Insulin Resistance Diet & Immune System Recovery Plan

universal. As befitting its nature, it is presented without assurance regarding its prolonged validity or interim quality. Trademarks that are mentioned are done without written consent and can in no way be considered an endorsement from the trademark holder.

BONUS:

As promised, please use your link below to claim your 3 FREE Cookbooks on Health, Fitness & Dieting Instantly

tiny.cc/q1u27y

You can also share your link with your friends and families whom you think that can benefit from the cookbooks or you can forward them the link as a gift!

Table of Contents

Insulin Resistance Diet Plan:

Guide on How to End Diabetes

Introduction

One in three Americans suffers from insulin resistance, most of them without knowing it. This includes over half of those over the age of 60 and an estimated 80% of those who are overweight. If unaddressed, insulin resistance can lead to Type 2 Diabetes and the negative health consequences associated with that, making them more susceptible to heart disease and strokes as well as causing nerve and kidney damage, robbing them of 10 years of life. Insulin resistance and Type 2 Diabetes have been on the rise over the last fifty years as diets have shifted to start including much more sugars and simple carbohydrates, especially from the over-processed foods that have become so common.

Thankfully, it can be reversed and this book provides a diet and lifestyle solutions that can help you reduce your insulin resistance and even reverse Type 2 Diabetes. The following chapters will provide an easy to understand overview of the causes and consequences of insulin resistance as well as how insulin works in the body. Building on this information, it provides easy to follow solutions that have been shown in research to lower insulin resistance and reverse Type 2 Diabetes. Finally, it will delve deeper into food, discussing the best foods to add to your diet for their known blood sugar lowering properties as well as providing a list of the foods that should be avoided at all costs. This look at food includes an in-depth but easy to understand explanation of nutrition labels and what to be on the lookout for when reading them.

Using the information provided by this book, you can start reducing your insulin resistance and lower your blood sugar levels today, but that is not all. Insulin resistance often comes with higher blood sugar levels that can cause fatigue and mental fogginess. By following the tips provided in the following chapters, your energy will return and your mind will sharpen. Don't suffer from insulin resistance for a day longer. Learn how you become insulin resistant and make the life-saving changes now.

Chapter 1: Understanding the Function of Insulin in the Body

Insulin is a hormone secreted by the pancreas that plays an instrumental and vital role in both human and animal metabolism. While it has other purposes as well, when it comes to metabolism, insulin controls the ability of cells to absorb glucose from the blood. This action regulates the blood sugar levels and in a person without type 2 diabetes or insulin resistance, this ensures that the level of glucose in the blood does not rise too high or fall too low. In order to better understand the function of insulin on the metabolism and how insulin resistance and diabetes can interfere with that function, a brief look into the metabolism is warranted. This will not be a deep dive into the science, just an easy to understand overview designed to give you the information that you will need in order to reverse insulin resistance and even diabetes.

How Humans Regularly Metabolize Food

The human body is a machine, much like the engine of a car. A car's engine powers the systems of the car that allow it to work. The human body is made of billions of cells that perform their specific purpose in order for the machine of man or woman to perform the background functions of life such as breathing, blood circulation, and neurons firing in the brain, as well as those functions under our control like movement. In order for a car to function, it needs fuel, internal combustion engines need gas, while electric cars need energy. The human body is no different and its cells get their fuel from the food that we eat namely carbohydrates, fats, proteins, and alcohol.

The human body can use any combination of fats, carbohydrates, proteins, and alcohol as fuel, but all organisms on the planet prefer glucose as fuel and human cells are no different. All of the cells of the body can run on glucose and it is their default fuel. Most carbohydrates are broken down into glucose and this moves directly into the bloodstream to be used by the cells as fuel. Some carbohydrates such as fructose have to be metabolized through the liver into glycogen which is then stored in the liver, as well as a small amount in the muscles to act as emergency fuel.

When the body ingests protein, it first converts the proteins into their component amino acids and then further metabolizes them into amino acids that can then be used to build up muscles or converted into glucose to be used as fuel. Fats are broken down in the stomach and absorbed in the small intestines. These broken down fats are then converted into energy for the muscle cells or stored in the antipode or fat cells for use later.

The human body lacks a mechanism for storing excess glucose for later use so any excess in glucose gets converted into fatty acids for storage in the fat cells. For modern humans with our easy access to calorie-dense foods full of carbohydrates that are easily converted into glucose, this has led to ever-rising obesity levels, insulin resistance, and diabetes, but looking at how human beings used to live shows that our metabolism is designed to allow us to survive long-term starvation and when simple carbohydrates like sugar were much rarer than today.

Early humans lived in what we now call a hunter-gatherer society. They ate the animals that they could catch and kill while supplementing the calories from hunting with foods they could gather from their surroundings such as berries, fruit, and nuts.

Hunters would often have to stalk their prey for days as they migrated through the early humans territory. Without ways to preserve food, it would have to be eaten soon after the kill in order to avoid it going bad. The human body's ability to store that food in the fat cells allowed it to take as much energy as it could in times that it had access to more calories and store it for when times were leaner.

How Human Metabolism Changes during Fasts, Starvation or Without Carbohydrates

While the cells of the human body prefer to use glucose or glycogen as their energy source, when the body does not receive any food energy either through a voluntary fast or involuntary starvation, it will have to convert some of its existing energy stored for use as fuel. As stated above, the body cannot store its preferred glucose for later use, instead, storing it as fatty acids in the antipode or fat cells. Once the body's glucose and glycogen are gone, the body begins to send signs to most of the cells to switch to using fatty acids from the antipode cells for energy and the liver begins to convert some of the fatty acids into ketone bodies in order to feed the brain.

The brain is of paramount importance to the body and uses up to a quarter of the background or basal metabolism. This is a much larger share of the metabolism than in any other animal. It also must be protected against diseases caused by bacteria and viruses. The mechanism of this protection is the blood-brain barrier. This prevents the movement of most compounds from the blood to the brain. Glucose is free to pass through as it fuels the brain. When the body is starved, the ketone bodies fuel the brain in lieu of glucose.

Before the starved body begins producing ketone bodies and the cells first start using the fatty acids in the antipode cells for energy, the liver and muscles emergency supply of glycogen are used for fuel. Generally, this stage of starvation lasts between two to three days though it differed from person to person and the body will convert the antipode cells into fuel exclusively for roughly a week. After that point, the body will begin to slowly break down the proteins that make up the skeletal muscles, the muscles that are used for movement.

The building of muscle cells requires the amino acids that make up proteins. If the body is not taking protein in, it cannot build muscles. In this context, building muscles is a much broader concept than the idea of building muscles in weightlifting or exercising. As a person moves, their muscles are subjected to wear and tear. This causes damage to the muscles that the body in the normal course would repair using the amino acids broken down from ingested protein. Without that food, the body will have to break down some muscle tissue in order to keep the muscles functioning properly.

This is a system that evolved to better serve our hunter-gatherer ancestors. They needed the ability to store as much energy as they could because there would often be prolonged periods of little to no calories. The system is forgiving of short fasts, where the body will use the fatty acids stored in the antipode cells for energy before being forced to cannibalize some of the muscle cells in order to use their protein to rebuild and fix strained muscles.

Similar to starvation or fasting, a diet that consists primarily of fat and protein with very little carbohydrates will force the body to use its stored fat as an energy source. Like with starvation, the body will use the stored glycogen in the liver and muscles as fuel for a couple of days and then turn to the stored fat in the antipode cells. By continuing to eat protein, the low carbohydrate diets avoid the loss in muscle mass as the consumed protein can be used to rebuild working muscles.

The Role of Insulin in Metabolizing Carbohydrates

After carbohydrates are consumed, they are broken down into glucose that the body moves into the bloodstream. This is the blood sugar level. When the blood sugar rises, insulin is released and it informs the cells that they should start taking in blood glucose for fuel and when they have the fuel they need, the insulin triggers the antipode cells to start converting excess blood sugar into fatty acids for long-term storage. Not all carbohydrates are the same when it comes to insulin rises.

Carbohydrates can generally be put into three different categories: simple, complex, and fiber. Simple carbohydrates are those that are more readily convertible into glucose by the body. All of the sugars are simple carbohydrates. Foods high in sugar, such as soda sweetened with High Fructose Corn Syrup or cane sugar and most packaged breakfast cereals are full of simple carbohydrates. Starchy carbohydrates such as vegetables and whole grains are examples of complex carbohydrates. Fiber is a carbohydrate that cannot be digested.

When the body consumes a simple carbohydrate, it is quickly converted into glucose either through the digestive tract or with some sugars such as fructose is converted into glycogen by the liver and becomes readily available to power the cells of the body and to be stored for later use in the fat cells. This causes a rapid rise in blood sugar and the pancreas responds with a spike in insulin to return the blood sugar back to normal. In addition to sugars, many complex carbohydrates can be turned into a simpler form that is quick to digest. Refined white flour is a good example of this. Flour comes from grains of wheat. A wheat grain includes the germ, the part of the seed that a new wheat plant would germinate from the endosperm, the stored nutrition the germ would use as it started to grow. These are covered by a hard protective covering called the bran. In refined white flour, the bran and germ are removed, leaving only the endosperm. Both the bran and germ are higher in fiber, protein, and fat than the endosperm. Whole wheat flour retains these parts of the grain which slows the release of insulin after consumption as the body needs more time to break it down into sugars.

Complex carbohydrates, on the other hand, need to be processed in order for the body to gain access to the sugars that it can convert to glucose. As this takes time, the glucose that the body converts from complex carbohydrates enters the bloodstream slowly. When consuming complex carbohydrates, the pancreas does not flood the bloodstream with insulin in a spike but releases insulin in smaller amounts to deal with the slow rise in the blood sugar. This gives the body more time to use the glucose converted from the food before the excess glucose is stored as fat.

When it comes to metabolism, fiber basically gets in the way but with positive consequences. Fibers cannot be converted into glucose to power the body, nor can it get converted into any other useful compound. Instead, it gets in the way of the body processing the carbohydrates it can convert into glucose. This slows the absorption of the glucose from the food, leading to a more gradual rise in blood sugar, reducing insulin spikes. It also takes up space in the stomach while the other carbohydrates are being broken down, lowering hunger.

Due to the subsidization of corn production in the United States, corn forms an abnormally large part of food in the food industry in the United States. As a consequence, high fructose corn syrup has become a standard sweetener in soft drinks and processed foods. In addition to the high fructose corn syrup, processed foods are often made using heavily refined carbohydrates, making most of the carbohydrates in these simple foods easily accessed by the body. Fructose, as stated above, must be processed by the liver into glycogen in order to be used by the body.

For our ancient hunter-gatherer ancestors, this caused few problems as fructose's main natural source was fruit, a limited aspect of the ancient diet. Before the cultivation of fruit, humans would only have access to the fruits and berries that grew naturally. One of the consequences of fruit agriculture was the increase in the sweetness of fruits. As humans began and continued to grow fruits, they crossbred them to contain more sugars. Even gorging on wild fruits and berries would have little effect on the livers of our ancient ancestors.

Today, due to its inexpensive nature, we have access to a gigantic amount of fructose, through high fructose corn syrup. As it was only synthesized in the 1970s, the long-term health effect of high fructose corn syrup is still being researched. Regardless of its possible negative effects in health, for the purpose of reducing insulin resistance, avoiding it is a good idea.

Chapter 2: What is Diabetes?

Diabetes is the name of three separate metabolic disorders, though only one type of diabetes, Diabetes Type 2 is the focus of this book. Type 1 Diabetes, more commonly known as juvenile diabetes, is an incurable condition where a person's body cannot create insulin at all. Sufferers of this form of diabetes must take insulin shots in order to survive. Gestational diabetes is similar to Type 2 Diabetes and effects between 2-10% of pregnant women.

The vast majority, up to 90% of people with diabetes have Type 2 Diabetes. In type 2 Diabetes, the body's cells have formed a resistance to insulin to the point where the pancreas cannot produce the required insulin to effectively lower the blood sugar level. This leads to higher levels of glucose in the blood which cause a variety of different serious health issues. For most who are diagnosed with Type 2 Diabetes, they built up a resistance to insulin over the years. Through proper diet and exercise, both insulin resistance and Type 2 diabetes are reversible. This will be covered in the next chapters.

Insulin Resistance

Insulin resistance is the precursor to Type 2 Diabetes. For many people who are prediabetic, there are few or no symptoms of insulin resistance, though others will exhibit the early symptoms of high blood sugar or hypoglycemia. The root cause of insulin resistance is related to food. Too many insulin spikes after the consumption of simple carbohydrates allow the cells to form a tolerance to insulin, similar to how some drugs such as opioids create a tolerance. With opioids, habitual users, both for pain management or recreational purposes, need to take more and more of the opioid in order to get the desired effect. Insulin resistance works the same way.

After receiving more and more insulin spikes, the cells start requiring more insulin when processing the glucose out of the blood. This raises the blood sugar level as the pancreas overworks to produce enough insulin to lower the level of sugar in the blood. As stated above, the body can't store this glucose and converts the excess into fatty acids stored in the fat cells. Weight gain and eventual obesity are often results of insulin resistance. Other symptoms could include an increase in thirst and hunger, weight gain (especially around the abdomen), increased blood pressure, sleepiness, depression, and mental strain including an inability to focus.

Insulin Resistance into Type 2 Diabetes

With more insulin spikes, the pancreas continues to overwork until it reaches the point where it cannot produce the amount of insulin to lower the blood sugar level to the normal amount. It is at this point that insulin resistance turns into Type 2 Diabetes. If simple carbohydrates are consumed in the same amounts as before, this will lead to extended periods of hypoglycemia or high blood sugar. The symptoms of hypoglycemia include an increase in thirst and hunger, frequent urination, blurred vision, weight loss, tingling feet and toes, dry and itchy skin, fatigue, and slow healing of wounds.

Chronic Type 2 Diabetes generally reduces life expectancy by about 10 years as hyperglycemia strains many systems of the body, including the heart and nerves. In addition, diabetes and obesity often go hand in hand, so the negative health consequences of both can compound.

Chapter 3: The Causes Behind Diabetes

For Type 2 Diabetes, the causes are primarily lifestyle in origin, though researchers have discovered over thirty different genes that are believed to influence the chances a person develops Type 2 Diabetes in their lifetime. Some of the genetic precursors are more common in some races than in others. Age also plays a part, with the development of Type 2 Diabetes later life more common than in youth, though rising obesity rates are making the development of Type 2 Diabetes earlier in life more common. Some researchers have found that sleep problems can also contribute to the development of Type 2 Diabetes.

Lifestyle Causes of Type 2 Diabetes

When it comes down to the development of Type 2 Diabetes, the most common cause is prolonged insulin resistance. As stated above, this is due to insulin spikes caused by the consumption of simple carbohydrates. In addition to the excess consumption of simple carbohydrates, a sedimentary lifestyle contributes as well. Without much movement or exercise, the body does not need to burn as many calories. The overconsumption of simple carbohydrates leads to the majority of those carbohydrates converted from glucose into fatty acids for storage in the fat cells leading to obesity.

This, in essence, forms a feedback loop. Eating more simple carbohydrates spikes both insulin and blood sugar levels, leading to greater insulin resistance as well as increases in the fat stores. As the person puts on more and more weight, they are often less active and their metabolism slows, converting more of their consumed carbohydrates into fat while increasing insulin resistance... until finally, they have developed Type 2 Diabetes.

More recently, researchers have begun to look to the impact a western diet might have on the gut flora and how these changes can affect insulin resistance. The human body contains several colonies of microorganisms that often provide benefits to the host human. Gut flora is the colonies living in the gastrointestinal system. While everyone's gut flora is different, studies have shown that those that eat a modern western diet, high in processed foods containing sugar and simple carbohydrates, and lacking in complex carbs and fiber, have a less diverse gut flora. Antibiotics can also change the makeup of the microorganisms in the gut.

The lack of diversity among gut flora has been shown to be a possible contributing factor towards developing obesity which makes insulin resistance and Type 2 Diabetes much more likely. There are several foods that contain live bacteria cultures or probiotics that can be eaten to re-diversify your gut flora. Cultured dairy products are most common in the western world. Yogurt, cultured buttermilk, and cheeses with live cultures such as some brie, gouda, and even higher quality cheddar cheeses contain probiotics. Fermented foods such as kimchee, sauerkraut, miso, and tempeh also contain probiotic microorganisms. Add some of these to your diet, as long as you are careful with the sugar content. Probiotic supplements are also available but remember that a lack of fiber and complex carbohydrates lead to a less diverse gut flora, so taking probiotics without adding more fiber and complex carbs to your diet will not sustain the probiotics in your gut.

Sleep might be an issue as well when it comes to the development of Type 2 Diabetes. Some research has shown that those with sleep issues are more likely to develop Type 2 Diabetes. These issues can include insomnia as well as just a lack of sleep. Everyone needs a different amount of sleep, so it is difficult to give an exact number, but most adults need between seven and nine hours of sleep per night. The quality of sleep might have an effect as well. Practicing good sleep hygiene can help prevent Type 2 Diabetes and improve your energy levels during the waking hours. Again, this is different for everyone, but most sleep is best in a cool, dark and quiet room.

Genetic Causes of Type 2 Diabetes

Currently, there are thirty-six identified genes that are believed to contribute to the possibility of developing Type 2 Diabetes some time in a person's life. Genetic predisposition is not the major factor in the development of Type 2 Diabetes but combined with a sedimentary lifestyle and obesity, they can greatly increase the risk.

There are genetic tests available to the general public that can show a person's predisposition. Doctors can perform these tests too. If diabetes is common in your family, it is possible that you have a genetic predisposition. Certain races are also more likely to develop Type 2 Diabetes. In the United States, the developments of Type 2 Diabetes as a percentage of adults by their race are as follows:

• Native American: 15%
• African American: 12.7%
• Hispanics: 12.1%
• Asians and Pacific Islanders: 8%
• Caucasians: 7.4%

The exact causes of this disparity are still being researched, but if you are a member of a higher risk race, ensuring that you minimize insulin resistance will only help to avoid developing Type 2

Diabetes.

Chapter 4: Natural Treatment for Diabetes

This chapter will explore the different natural treatments for reducing insulin resistance and reversing Type 2 Diabetes. Diet plays a large part in this, and this chapter will provide information on several different types of diets that have been shown to help reduce insulin resistance and reverse diabetes. Each of these diets has their pros and cons when it comes to their power in reversing insulin resistance. Some of them are more restrictive and will provide a much stronger insulin resistance reducing effect while others are more gradual.

In addition to diet, exercise, and stress reduction have been shown to have an effect on insulin resistance and Type 2 Diabetes. This chapter will provide several strategies to increase your physical exertion to reduce insulin resistance. For the exercise-phobic, small changes can lead to greater effects later and if you combine even the smallest increase in exercise with one of the diets discussed in the diet section, you will most likely find that your energy levels will quickly increase. Insulin resistance can lead to fatigue and longer recovery time from physical exertion. Some of the low carb and intermittent fasting diets can stabilize insulin levels within a few days, leading to an almost immediate boost in energy.

Just as we, modern humans have an almost immediate access to a vast amount of simple calories were our ancient ancestors had little, the modern world adds a great deal of stress that our ancestors rarely had to worry about. We increasingly live our lives by the clock, scheduling more and more of our precious time with deadlines and other commitments. That stress can lead to insulin resistance and Type 2 Diabetes. In addition to diet and exercise, this chapter will briefly touch on some simple ways to reduce your stress.

Diet and Insulin Resistance

When it comes to reducing insulin resistance and even reversing Type 2 Diabetes, diet is 90% of the solution. This makes sense as a diet high in simple carbohydrates is the cause of 99% of Type 2 Diabetes. This section will compare and contrast several different diets that have been shown to be helpful in reducing insulin resistance, including a couple that has been shown in research studies to actually reverse diabetes. The diets that fall into the latter category are more restrictive about carbohydrates, but in addition to their reduction of insulin resistance, they can provide a multitude of other benefits.

The traditional modern medical diabetic diet focuses on eating more complex carbohydrate such as whole grains, legumes, and vegetables while avoiding simple carbohydrates such as sugar, processed foods, and refined grains. This, combined with moderate exercise can manage Type 2 Diabetes and will help to lower insulin resistance, but it will likely do so at a glacial pace and some complex carbs are better than others when it comes to reversing Type 2 Diabetes and reducing insulin resistance. The next chapter will discuss this in much more detail.

The glycemic index can be a powerful tool that can help you determine the best complex carbohydrates to eat as part of your insulin resistance reducing diet. The glycemic index is a chart that measures the effect a certain food has on a person's blood sugar level and compares that to glucose. Foods that are high on the glycemic index will cause steeper insulin spikes as they are more easily converted to glucose. Foods on the lower end lead to a gradual release of insulin as the complex starches and fiber filled foods are slowly broken down into glucose.

The amount and type of cooking can change the glycemic index of the food as well. Take the potato for example. Potatoes tend to be high on the glycemic index, usually between 60 and 90. Mashed and boiled potatoes usually have a higher glycemic index compared to french fried potatoes. This is caused by the cooking method. Boiling potatoes take a lot longer than frying and in the long cooking time, more of the complex starches are broken down into simpler carbohydrates that the body can more readily convert into glucose. Along the same lines, al dente pasta has a lower glycemic index than fully cooked or softer pasta. The cooking process breaks down some of the starches in the noodles.

One final note about the glycemic index, at least in this chapter, is to remember that most glycemic index calculations are specific to the serving size. For example, lentils are quite low on the glycemic index, usually around 30. This is for a 150 gram or 1 cup serving. A larger serving will likely have a greater effect on blood sugar and therefore rising insulin levels than a smaller serving.

The traditional modern medical diet for Type 2 Diabetes and insulin resistance on focusing on more complex carbohydrates is better used by those that seek to prevent insulin resistance and Type 2 Diabetes. For those who are already heavily resistant to insulin or have been diagnosed with Type 2 Diabetes, low carb diets will provide much more benefits often quite quickly.

Low Carbohydrate Diets for Reducing Insulin Resistance and Reversing Type 2 Diabetes

The understanding of the process in which insulin is released from the pancreas and its role in the regulation of blood sugar levels is a relatively new finding. Insulin was first discovered in the mid 19th century but it was not extracted and purified until the 1920s. Prior to that, the treatment for Type 2 Diabetes was a low to no carb diet. Outside of this context, a no carb diet was considered by the medical mainstream of the time to be insufficient for humans. An explorer of the Canadian Arctic by the name of Vilhjalmur Stefansson was the first to advocate a meat-centered diet in the early 20th century.

Stefansson as an Arctic explorer spent a great deal of time in the far north and had observed the Inuit, the Native Americans that live year-round above the Arctic Circle and their peculiar diet. The Inuit in the far north had little access to agriculture as there are no crops that can be grown in such cold environments and survive the extended period of darkness that engulfs the North for half the year. The Inuit's only non-meat sources of food were the few gathered berries and plants that grew in the less harsh summer months as well as seaweeds. Outside of this, they ate exclusively from marine mammals like whales, walruses, and seals as well as arctic land mammals such as caribou and polar bears.

The breakdown of the Inuit's diet generally consisted of fifty percent of their calories from fat, thirty-five percent protein and only fifteen percent from carbohydrates. Sea mammals tend to have large stores of fat to insulate their warm-blooded bodies from the frigid temperatures of the Arctic Sea so it is understandable that the Inuit's diet consists of so much fat. Stefansson like other polar explorers would journey with a large amount of western food, primarily canned meats and vegetables as well as hardtack, a type of simple hard cracker that was common rations for long sea journeys and military campaigns in the past.

On one of his journeys to the North, Stefansson's team lost a lot of their supplies and they adopted a more Inuit diet, harvesting seals and walruses to survive. He found that he could thrive on such a diet and brought his findings back to New York where they were panned by the medical establishment. To prove his findings, Stefansson adopted a meat only diet for an entire year while under medical supervision. His no carb diet is well beyond the more popular low carb diets of today, as he ate one hundred percent meat products getting all the requisite vitamins and minerals required to survive from beef kidneys and other organ meat. In the end, he was perfectly healthy eating no carbs.

Low carb diets languished in medical obscurity after that until the 1970s when Robert Atkins formulated his Atkins Diet. This diet advocated a short period of almost no carbohydrates and then gradually increasing carbohydrates to the diet until the weight loss goal is achieved. At that point, the dieter would maintain the weight by eating a moderately low carb diet. As with Stefansson, generations earlier, the conventional medical authorities discounted Atkin's low carbohydrate diet. The preferred diet at the time reduced fat consumption and favored carbohydrates. The Atkins diet gained greater popularity in the early 2000s and while it is not as popular as it was a decade ago, it brought low carb diets into the mainstream. Other low carb diets have followed and today there is a multitude of low carb diet friendly processed and frozen foods available though they are often expensive and low carb dieters are often better off without them.

Atkin's Diet

While not as popular as it was during its peak in the early 2000s, the Atkin's diet is still one of the more popular low carb diet options and it can be used to reduce insulin resistance and reverse Type 2 Diabetes. The Atkin's Diet is split into four separate phases. Induction, Balancing, Pre-Maintenance, and Maintenance. The first phase is especially helpful for battling insulin resistance as it restricts carbs to only 20 grams a week. Each successive phase increases the amount of carbs. Under the Atkin's Diet rules, fiber does not count as carbs for determining the level of carbs you can eat as fiber cannot be digested and will not raise blood sugar levels, resulting in a rise in insulin.

If you are considering a very low carb diet such as Atkins, remember that not all carbs are the same and for reducing insulin resistance this is especially important. A single slice of white bread contains 20 grams of carbohydrates as does a large plate of leafy green vegetables. Consuming a single slice of bread will spike insulin much higher than eating a plate full of leafy green vegetables. When looking for carbs to eat in a low carb diet, refer to the glycemic index and stick with carbs that are on the lowest section at least under 50. This will ensure that your carb intake will have little effect on raising your blood sugar.

The Atkin's diet recommends staying at the induction phase where you restrict carbs to below 20 grams for at least two weeks. Should you choose, you can continue on longer than those two weeks in the induction phase. This can supercharge weight loss as it puts the body into ketosis. As explained in greater detail in the first chapter, when the body is starved, the body lives off of the glycogen stored in the liver and skeletal muscles before turning to the stored fat cells, converting the fatty acids stored there into energy for the cells of the body. By removing almost all carbohydrates from the diet, the body is starved of foods that it can easily convert into glucose. In essence, this tricks the body into thinking it is starving so that it uses the fat stores for fuel. As long as the dieter takes in a sufficient amount of protein, the body will not have to cannibalize the muscle tissue in order to get access to more amino acids.

While you move from the induction phase of Atkins, beware of the type of carbs that you add to your diet and the amounts. For reducing insulin resistance, stick to carbs that are low on the glycemic index. Vegetables are one of the best sources of carbs early in these diets, and as a general rule, leafy vegetables are lower than non-leafy vegetable on the index and those that grow above the ground are lower than those that grow under the ground. Vegetables also contain a great deal of fiber that will help to slow any rise in insulin levels. Most beans are on the lower side of the glycemic index and many of them are high in protein and fiber as well. Note that canned beans are often much higher on the glycemic index than dried beans.

Ketogenic Diet

The ketogenic diet is similar to the induction phase of the Atkin's Diet where carbs are severely restricted so that the body remains in ketosis. Most proponents of ketogenic diets do not differentiate between what fats and proteins are consumed and generally favor a higher fat to protein ratio. For reversing Type 2 Diabetes and reducing insulin resistance, however, the choice of fats can be important. Trans fats such as margarine or any fat labeled 'hydrogenated' or 'partially hydrogenated' should be avoided. These are unsaturated fats that have been saturated with a hydrogen atom for stabilization and preservation purposes and they used to be quite common in processed foods. In the last 20 years as they became better understood, the health risks posed by them have caused many governments to ban their addition to processed foods. They are known to lead to obesity and are thought to contribute to Type 2 Diabetes, though that connection is unproven. Regardless of your Type 2 Diabetes risk, avoiding trans fats is a good idea.

Remaining in ketosis is important in a ketogenic diet, both for maximizing weight loss as well as lowering insulin resistance and reversing Type 2 Diabetes. There are several products on the market that can be used to determine if you are in ketosis. Ketone bodies change a person's breath, adding a fruity and often nail-polish-remover-like scent. There are Ketone breath analyzers that can be purchased at many stores or online. Ketosis can also be determined by analyzing urine. Ketosis strips can be used like pregnancy tests to determine if your body is in ketosis. As you add small amounts of carbs into your ketogenic diet, use products such as these to determine if the added carbs have taken you out of ketosis.

Paleo Diet

The Paleo diet is a more recent low carb diet fad that attempts to mimic the type of diet our ancient ancestors ate when living as hunter-gatherers. This hunter-gatherer diet removes all carbs except those that the ancients would have been able to forage from their environment. This includes berries, nuts, fruits, and some vegetables. Along with these 'foraged' foods, meat and seafood are freely eaten. For reducing insulin resistance and reversing Type 2 Diabetes, this diet might not work depending on the amount and type of fruits and berries eaten. While our ancestors ate these foods freely, their access to them was quite limited so they made up a small part of their diet.

For a person suffering from insulin resistance or Type 2 Diabetes, a large number of fruits and berries will cause insulin spikes, reducing the effectiveness of the diet in reducing insulin resistance. Should you desire to go paleo, use the glycemic index or even stick with the Atkin's or Ketogenic diet's restrictions on carbs to ensure that you get the maximum reduction to insulin resistance.

General Tips for Low Carb Diets and Reducing Insulin Resistance

Regardless of the type of low carb diet that you choose, there are a couple of important things to keep in mind. Unless you are like Stefansson and are eating a lot of organ meats, a low carb diet can be deficient on some vital nutrients such as Vitamin C. Taking a vitamin supplement while eating a low carb diet is essential to avoid scurvy or rickets. Eating a fair amount of leafy vegetables will provide more vital nutrients than meat and fat alone, but a supplement will ensure that you get the required vitamins and minerals.

Another less common but potentially serious issue is protein poisoning or rabbit starvation. This is caused by a low carb diet that does not include enough fat and named rabbit starvation because rabbits are an extremely lean meat. If one attempts to eat rabbit alone after a week or so, they will experience increased bouts of diarrhea, fatigue, headaches, and an insatiable hunger. Stefansson experienced this on one of his Arctic expeditions. A low carb diet without fat will bring on rabbit starvation so make sure to include a fair share of fat in your low carb diet. This will likely not be an issue for most as it is quite easy to eat fat while low carb dieting.

Intermittent Fasting for Reducing Insulin Resistance

One of the newest entries in the diet world is Intermittent Fasting. Fasting, abstaining from food for a short period of time has been a part of human culture since prehistory and is still practiced to some extent in several major world religions. For probationers of Islam for example, fasting during the daylight hours of the holy month of Ramadan is a religious obligation and short fasts are common in several orthodox Christian faiths as well as in several eastern faiths. As discussed in the first chapter, during fasts and starvation, the body uses up the glycogen stored in the liver and skeletal muscles before turning to the fatty acids stored in the fat cells as an energy source. Intermittent fasting uses this mechanism for weight loss purposes and general health.

When it comes to intermittent fasting for reducing insulin resistance and reversing Type 2 Diabetes, it is most effective when combined with a low carb diet, though using an intermittent fasting method with a carb friendly diet that focuses on foods lower on the glycemic index will also be able to provide a reduction in insulin resistance. For those who do not suffer from insulin resistance or Type 2 Diabetes, an unrestricted intermittent fasting program can be effective in preventing their onset, but ineffective in reversing Type 2 Diabetes.

There are several versions of intermittent fasting that range from short daily fasts days where very little calories to no calories are consumed. These can be combined for greater effects. The following section will briefly describe a few of the more popular intermittent fasting methods and finish with an example of how to combine them as well as start on intermittent fasting program in a gradual way. An extra caution for women, there are biological differences between men and women that can make fasting more difficult for women and can lead to some negative side effects, specifically regarding their reproductive system. Women who want to experiment with intermittent fasting should be cautious and approach it slowly, especially if they want children in the future.

With any kind of intermittent fasting, water and unsweetened tea, and coffee during the fasts are always allowed and you should make sure to remain hydrated. Vigorous exercise during fasting periods especially as you start your fasting regimen is not recommended. Keep any exercise low-impact and save the more strenuous exercises for periods when you are eating.

16:8 Intermittent Fasting

The 16:8 intermittent fast is one of the easiest to perform. This is a daily fast where you abstain from eating 16 hours of the day while eating during the other 8. As most people sleep an average of 8 hours a day, half of the fast happens while you sleep, adding to its ease. One of the more common eating periods is noon to 8 pm, but the actual period used varies amongst the dieter. Some people prefer the early morning calorie boost and shift the eating window earlier, while others prefer a later dinner and shift it to as late as 3 pm.

This fast has been shown to reduce insulin resistance even when the eating period is not limited as to carbs or sugars, but even when not eating a low carb diet avoiding simple carbs and sugars in the first meal of the day will provide a greater reduction in insulin resistance.

During the fasting period, the body will use what glucose it has on hand from your last meal before switching to the glycogen in the liver and skeletal muscles. This will cause a drop in insulin levels even among the most insulin resistant. A post fast meal high in sugars or simple carbohydrates will cause an insulin spike and higher blood sugar levels.

While most proponents of 16:8 advocates use it daily, for a more gradual introduction, eat 16:8 two to three days a week for the first two weeks. Make sure that these days are spaced with normal eating days between them to make it even easier to follow. Add a 16:8 day each week after until you are eating 16:8 every day. At this point, you will be in the habit and more likely to continue. The 16:8 fast will help reduce insulin resistance even when you have a cheat day and eat too much sugar or simple carbs. Just try and keep them rare and hop back on the wagon the next day, or even use a more severe fast the day after to get your body back to its fat burning state.

5:2 Method

In this intermittent fasting method, the ratio refers to fasting days and normal eating days. In 5:2, you eat normally for five days out of the week while restricting yourself to only 500 calories on two non-consecutive days of the week. This can be combined with a low-carb diet, though for hunger sating on the 500 calorie days, leafy vegetables, as well as low glycemic index beans and grains, will help keep hunger at bay. Beef and chicken broths are recommended on fast days as well, but be cautious of the sodium level.

As with the 16:8 methods, the 5:2 can be approached more gradually by starting with a single fasting day or even starting with a more gradual fasting level. Reduce your calories on the chosen fasting day to 1000 for two weeks before moving down to 500. Add a second day of the week to this regimen and move to the 5:2 method.

On the five-eating days, sticking with a 16:8 eating habit will provide even more insulin resistance reducing effect. The daily fasting period will lead to a lower starting blood sugar level when you eat your first meal of the day. This has the additional benefit of allowing your 16:8 eating pattern to better become a habit.

Eat-Stop-Eat Method

With the Eat Stop Eat method, we have reached the more extreme intermittent fast. This advocates a single 24-hour period of fasting during the week. A fast that begins after a big dinner on the night before and ends with a dinner the next day is the most common form of the Eat Stop Eat method, though as with other intermittent fasts, it is up to the dieter to determine when to best start their fast. One of the other benefits of starting after a big dinner is that it makes the fast more comparable with the 16:8 method.

A 24 hour fast can be too much for some people and can cause headaches as well as dizziness and irritability. It is best to work into a fast such as this by sticking to a 16:8 for several weeks before adding a 5:2 style 500 calorie fast day for a few more weeks and then reducing the calories on the fast day to zero. As with other intermittent fasts, staying hydrated during the fast day is important. Water, unsweetened tea, and coffee can be consumed as you like.

Alternate Day Fasting

The most extreme of the intermittent fasting methods discussed in this book, Alternate Day Fasting is exactly what it sounds like. You eat normally for a day and then do not eat at all the next day, repeating this pattern every two days. This can provide amazing insulin resistance reduction, especially when combined with a low carb diet, but can be extremely difficult to stick with. Modifying this method by substituting the 500 calorie days of the 5:2 method can make it easier to stick with. In the end, the dieter can discover the best method of intermittent fasting for their own body and lifestyle.

Exercise to Help Reduce Insulin Resistance

Exercise is often paired with diet changes in doctor's recommendations for those suffering from insulin resistance and even Type 2 Diabetes. While in reality, it forms a much smaller part of the solution than diet, paired together with a low carb or at least low simple carb and sugar diet, exercise will help bring your blood sugar levels back to normal levels. This section will explore adding exercise to your diet to maximize benefits. This section will be geared more towards those who do not regularly exercise as opposed to those who already have an exercise regiment. If you already exercise regularly, keep it up and look to the end of the sections for tips about exercising on a low carb diet to ensure that you get the most benefit from both exercise and diet

Adding More Activity to Your Life

For most of us who have issues with insulin resistance, leading a sedentary lifestyle is one of the factors that led us into this state. As you remove sugars and simple carbohydrates from your diet, you will alleviate some of the symptoms of high blood sugar as you will not be spiking your insulin levels in the same way. This will likely increase your energy, doubly so if you stick with a ketogenic low carb diet. This returning energy can be used to add more activity to your life.

Obesity and insulin resistance create a feedback loop of a sort. As you overindulge in sugars and simple carbohydrates, you pack on extra pounds while your cells become more resistant to insulin. Your blood sugar rises and this adds to your fatigue, leading to less activity. In the end, this slows your metabolism and makes it even easier for you to gain even more weight. A low carb diet, as well as one that avoids sugars and simple carbs, will help alleviate this fatigue. Adding more activity into your life even at an incremental and slow pace will help to establish a positive feedback loop. As your energy increases because of your diet, you will find adding activity to your life easier and your motivation higher.

For those who do not regularly exercise, the goal at the beginning of your plan to reduce your insulin resistance is to increase your activity by a small amount. As you stick with an insulin resistance reducing diet, you will likely find yourself with more and more energy, leading to increased levels of activity later. But as a start, you can take it slow, finding ways to add a little extra movement to your day.

A pedometer, or even a pedometer app for your phone, can be very beneficial in tracking your activity level and adding to it. These track the amount of steps you have taken in a day and the phone apps often track the distance walked as well. In order to get the best out of one of these pedometers, use it to track your steps each day for a week to determine your general activity amount before adding more.

The next step is to look at your day and try to find places and times you can add a little extra movement. One of the first targets should be any extended time sitting down. For many, this is unavoidable. So many of us have jobs where we sit in front of a computer screen multiple hours of the day and after working all day, decompress in front of the TV with our family. While sitting for a long time might be unavoidable, you can break it up with short periods of activity. Even two to five minutes of movement an hour will make a difference at the start of your insulin resistance reducing regimen. Set a timer on your phone for an hour while at work or vegging out in front of the TV. Once it goes off, stand up, stretch out, and take a quick walk to the water cooler, kitchen, break room, etc.

For those who drive often, there are some simple ways to add more steps by parking in different places. Whenever you go to the grocery store, park further away from the store. If you do not have assigned parking at work, park further from the door. If your trip will take you to multiple places that are not too far apart, park at one of them and walk to the others. Adding small ankle or arm weights while you walk can further boost the benefit you get out of your increased activity. These small steps will add up and as your energy levels rise, you will be ready and willing to add a bit more activity.

Adding Exercise to Your Insulin Resistance Reducing Diet

As you progress and want to start adding more activity to your routine, there are several things that you should keep in mind. Exercise causes wear and tear to your muscles and you need to have a steady stream of protein coming into your body through food in order for your muscles to heal and rebuild. If you are not taking in enough protein, your body will have to cannibalize your muscle cells for the amino acids needed for those repairs. The good news is that following a low carb diet will almost guarantee that you get enough protein. It is possible to not eat enough protein by simply avoiding sugars and simple carbs, but outside some vegetarians, this is also unlikely. If you are a vegetarian or want to eat a vegetarian diet, make sure you get enough protein.

Hydration is equally important. As you exercise, make sure to drink enough water. Strenuous exercise can lead to a loss of hydration through sweat and your body needs water. Make sure to be properly hydrated before you exercise, while you do it and afterward as well. As you will be following a diet that avoids sugars, sugary drinks should be avoided as hydration sources. Water is your best bet.

When it comes to the type of exercises, there are basically two different types - aerobic and anaerobic. Aerobic exercises raise the heart rate for an extended period of activity. Running, biking and walking are examples of aerobic exercises. Anaerobic exercise, on the other hand, is short and intense exercise. Weightlifting is the standard example of anaerobic exercise though interval training and short sprints are also anaerobic exercises. Both types can play an important role in reducing insulin resistance.

With aerobic exercise, it is important to have a short warm up and cool down period bookending the greater exertion of the exercise. Take five minutes to stretch and walk before jogging or walking more briskly. Afterward, slow down and continue to walk slowly for five minutes. This prepares the body for the exercise, leading to less strain and similarly allows the body to slowly return to less activity reducing muscle stress.

Weight training can be an effective tool in boosting your metabolism, even if you do not desire large or bulging muscles.

Working your muscles requires fuel for the muscle cells, fuels they get from the blood sugar, lowering its level. Larger muscles burn more fuel even when they are not in use, leading to a rise in your metabolic rate. Resistance training, using bands or weights can be particularly helpful in strengthening muscles and increasing endurance. When choosing a resting training regimen, make sure to rotate the muscle groups and not exercise the same groups in successive days. This will give your muscles time to recover preventing muscle strain.

Lowering Stress to Aid in Reducing Insulin Resistance

Stress can almost be an inescapable part of life in the modern world and that excess stress can contribute to insulin resistance and Type 2 Diabetes at least indirectly. Stress can contribute to poor eating, pushing people to eat sugary snacks or cheat on their diet. Stress can lead to depression as well, sapping motivation. Mindfulness exercises, a form of short meditation have been shown to be effective on curbing excess stress.

Some mindfulness exercises can be combined with exercising. Practicing yoga can be a form of mindfulness exercise and you can also perform a walking meditation. While in a brief walk, clear your mind beforehand with a couple of deep and slow breaths. Focus on the sensation of breathing, in and out, in and out. Start to walk focusing on the sensation of your feet hitting the ground with each step. As you continue to walk, slowly move your focus upward through your legs, torso, and arms and finally focusing on the senses, the smells, feel of the cool, or hot air on your face, and the sounds around you. A five-minute walking meditation can help melt the stress away.

Turn your meals into meditations as well where you have the chance. Like everything else in the modern world, we often eat on the run. When you can, eat your meal slowly and focus fully on the sensation of eating at least with the first few bites. Think about the textures and flavors you taste and the sensation of chewing and swallowing. Not only this will curb stress, but eating slower has been shown to have an effect on the amount a person eats. You are more likely to eat less when you eat slower, as the signals in the stomach that tells your brain it is full take a few minutes to come into effect, minutes you could have been overeating.

Mindfulness exercises are not for everyone, but they can be powerful tools to reduce stress. If the few discussed above are not your style, there are plenty more that you can discover on the internet and in books dedicated to meditation and mindfulness. Ultimately, if you are overstressed, you are the best person to determine what works for reducing your own stress. Whatever that is, do it… as long as it isn't binging on sugary snacks!

Chapter 5: Eating for Lower Blood Sugar Levels

The types and amounts of different foods consumed, specifically sugars and simple carbohydrates are the primary cause of insulin resistance and Type 2 Diabetes. Unsurprisingly, a diet that avoids sugars and simple carbohydrates are also the keys to reducing insulin resistance and reversing Type 2 Diabetes. While different diets useful in controlling blood sugar spikes were discussed in the last chapter, this chapter will delve much deeper into food when seeking to reduce insulin resistance.

The chapter will start with an in-depth look at the glycemic index and how you use it to choose foods that will minimize blood sugar spikes. This will include a look at foods that are known to fight insulin resistance as well as those that should be avoided the most. From there, it will move into a discussion of nutrition labels to give you all the information you need to quickly determine the effect that food will have on your blood sugar, as well as your net carbs if you are going low carb.

Glycemic Index and Glycemic Load

The previous chapter briefly touched on the concept of the glycemic index, the chart that compares the effect on blood sugar a given food will have to that of glucose. Glucose is given a glycemic index of 100 and foods that fall below 50 glycemic index are considered low GI foods. Those between 50 and 70 are Medium GI, whole foods with scores above 70 are high GI foods. For the purpose of preventing insulin resistance and Type 2 Diabetes, sticking to foods that are in the low and medium range is often sufficient, but for those who want to reduce existing insulin resistance and reverse Type 2 Diabetes, it is best to stick to foods on the lower end of the chart.

For most foods, the glycemic index provides enough information, but it can be used in conjunction with the glycemic load to better determine the effect that a specific amount of food will have on your blood sugar. A single unit of glycemic load is roughly equivalent to the effect of a single gram of glucose. To determine the glycemic load, there is a little math involved but we will walk through it slowly, with multiple examples, to allow even the most math-phobic among you to understand.

Step 1: Determine the glycemic index of the food in question. Here, the internet will be your ally as several sites contain glycemic indexes for most common foods. www.glycemicindex.com is a good site that not only includes both glycemic index and load of common foods but also calculates them for pre-packaged foods.

Step 2: With the glycemic index number of the food, the next step is to determine the carbs in the serving size. For many foods, this can be determined by looking at the nutritional information provided on the package. Be aware, however, that many packaged foods list a smaller serving size than the average person would eat. Look at the label under carbs. Take the total number of carbs in grams and subtract the grams of fiber from that number. Fiber is indigestible so it does not count towards net carbs. If you are looking at a single serving according to the package, move on to the next step. If you need to determine the glycemic load of multiple servings, multiply the net carbs by the number of servings.

Step 3: Multiply the net carbs in the amount of the food by the glycemic index and then divide that number by 100. This is the glycemic load.

Examples are often the best way for people to understand the math. A single slice of white bread weighs about 30 grams and contains 14 grams of net carbohydrates. It is a 71 in the glycemic index. 71 x 14 = 980 and 980 / 100 = 9.8 meaning that a single slice of bread has a glycemic load of 9.8. The glycemic load for two slices of bread would use the same formula with double the net carbs, so 71 x 28 (14 x 2) = 1,988. 1,988 / 100 = 19.88.

Some foods are deceptively high on the Glycemic index because it does not factor in the amount of carbs. Watermelon is an example of this. A 120 gram serving of watermelon has a glycemic index of 80 but it is mostly water so it only has 6 grams of net carbs per a 120-gram serving. 80 x 6 = 480. 480 / 100 = 4.8. So while watermelon is a high glycemic index food, its glycemic index is relatively low.

Other foods tend towards the reverse. Whole wheat spaghetti is a good example. A 180 gram serving of whole wheat spaghetti has a glycemic index of 37, pretty low, but it contains 36 grams of net carbs. 37 x 36 = 1,332. 1,332 / 100 = 13.32, in the middle ground of glycemic loads.

For the purpose of lowering insulin resistance and reversing Type 2 Diabetes, glycemic loads below 10 are preferred while those above 15 should be avoided. For the greatest effect, the following guidelines should be followed. For foods that have a glycemic index of 50 or below, avoid foods that have a glycemic load above 10. For foods that have a glycemic index above 50, avoid those that have a glycemic load above 5.

Dieters using a low carb diet to remain in ketosis should choose foods that have even lower numbers on the glycemic index and load when choosing to add foods that contain carbohydrates to their diet. Add foods that have a glycemic index of 40 or lower as long as their glycemic load is under 8 and for foods that have a glycemic index of 40 or more, only add foods with a glycemic load under 4. This will ensure that any rise in blood sugar from the added carbohydrates will be gradual, avoiding an insulin spike. Adding these carbs as part of a meal that includes fiber, protein, and fat as well will further slow insulin spikes.

Foods that Help Reduce Insulin Resistance

While the above information concerning the glycemic index and load can be used to generally find the best types of foods to reduce insulin resistance, there are also some specific foods that contain specific nutrients that have been shown to reduce insulin resistance. These nutrients include anti-antioxidants, Omega 3 Oils, and herbs and spices with insulin-like effects that can lower blood sugar.

Herbs and spices are of particular note as they are packed with flavors while having few, if any, calories. One of the major issues people have with sticking to a diet is boredom. With low carb diets, you can eat a lot of meats and in carb friendly diets, low glycemic index foods such as lentils and quinoa, but that can become repetitive. Herbs and spices can be used to alter the flavors and make a routine meal exotic. Basil, used extensively in Italian and Thai cuisine, can have a blood sugar lowering effect as can cumin and turmeric, common spices in curries. Cinnamon is another spice with insulin-like effects. Stevia is a recent plant derived calorie-free sweetener and can be used to indulge your sweet tooth on occasion without cheating too badly.

Omega-3 fatty acids are a crucial nutrient that has been shown to have a positive impact with a host of different health problems. They lower triglyceride levels in the blood, reducing the risk of heart disease, they can help with joint movement for those that suffer from arthritis and might even lower the risk of depression. There is also some evidence that they can assist in reducing insulin resistance. Fatty fish such as salmon, tuna, and sardines are great sources for omega 3s as are nuts. Omega 3s are also available in supplement form and more recently, eggs that are high in omega 3s have become commonly available. These are laid by chickens fed with a high Omega 3 diet. All of these foods are great for low carb and carb friendly insulin resistant reducing diets.

Antioxidants are compounds that inhibit oxidation. Oxidation of steel creates rust and corrosion. Inside the body, oxidation leads to the production of free radicals that can bind to DNA as well as proteins. This results in cell damage. Some of the complications of diabetes, such as nerve damage involve oxidation caused by free radicals. Adding antioxidants to the diet can help to reverse this damage as insulin resistance is lowered. Several fruits and berries are high in antioxidants such as blueberries, strawberries, raspberries, and grapes. Dark chocolate has high levels as well. These foods should be added in moderation as they all contain sugars and will lead to blood sugar spikes should they be consumed in excess. Less sugary foods high in antioxidants include dark green vegetables, nuts, and sweet potatoes.

Probiotics are also a potential reducing superfood for insulin resistance. The human body is teeming with different colonies of microorganisms such as bacteria, viruses, and even fungi. In fact, there are three times as many cells in these colonies than there are human cells in the body. For the most part, these colonies of microorganisms are beneficial. When it comes to insulin resistance, the most important colonies of microorganisms in the human body are the gut flora. From the name you likely guessed where these colonies live, in the gastrointestinal tract. As briefly discussed in chapter three, a western diet high in sugars and other simple carbs but lacking in fiber and complex carbohydrates can lead to a less diverse gut flora that can contribute to obesity as well as insulin resistance and Type 2 Diabetes.

Several foods are available that contain probiotic live cultures and probiotic supplements are available as well. In order to get the most benefit from these probiotics, increasing the amount of fiber and complex carbohydrates in the form of leafy vegetables will help feed your new gut flora. Cultured dairy products such as yogurt and buttermilk are sources for probiotics as well as some cheeses. Higher quality brie, gouda, and cheddar are good cheeses to find probiotics. Fermented products are another source of probiotics, this can include kimchee, sauerkraut, miso, and tempeh. When looking to add some of these products to your diet, be cautious of the carb and sugar content. Kimchee and sauerkraut do contain a little sugar as can miso.

Foods That Cause Insulin Spikes

By now, you are likely familiar with the foods that you need to avoid - sugars and simple carbohydrates. This section will look at some specific foods that are packed with sugars and other simple carbohydrates that cause the largest insulin spikes. Ideally, these foods should be avoided completely, at least until you have normalized your insulin resistance, and even then they are best in moderation. If you do consume them, do so sparingly and at the same time that you eat other less likely foods to spike your blood sugar. Take white rice for example. The Japanese often eat white rice with only furikake, a spice mixture of fish, seaweed, sesame seeds, sugar, and salt. Eating this would result in an insulin spike. Eating the same amount of rice, topped with stir-fried beef and broccoli would result in a more gradual rise in insulin as the beef and broccoli would slow the absorption. Just make sure not to use a high sugar sauce!

The foods that create the largest insulin spikes are sugary soft drinks. These are basically just sugar in water and lead to an immediate spike in insulin. Given their inexpensive nature and availability in large sizes, it is incredibly easy to overindulge in sugary soft drinks. A can of cola is a 63 on the glycemic index and contains 42 grams of sugar. 63 x 42 = 2,646 / 100 = a glycemic load of 26.46. A 22 oz. bottle has a glycemic load of 41.58. That is the equivalent of eating 41.58 grams of glucose and a huge insulin spike. Diet sodas can be used as a substitute, but there is some evidence that artificial sweeteners can cause small insulin spike themselves, albeit without a rise in blood sugar. Water is a better alternative and for those that prefer bubbles in their water, seltzers flavored with a small amount of lemon or lime juice are an excellent alternative to soda.

Other non-liquid sweets such as pastries, candies, and sugary cereals are also high on the list of things to avoid entirely. This can be difficult for those with a sweet tooth. A small amount of dark chocolate can sate the chocoholics and there are sugar-free candies on the market that use sugar alcohols instead of sugar as a sweetener. Sugar alcohols offer sweetness without the blood sugar spike of regular sugars but they have their own drawbacks.

Consumed in excess, sugar alcohols can have a pronounced laxative effect. The exact amount of sugar alcohols that cause the laxative effect differs person to person, so they are best used sparingly when you have a particular craving.

The final area of foods that you should generally avoid entirely is refined carbohydrates and processed foods. When grains such as rice and wheat are refined, the more fibers parts of the grain are removed, leaving the easier to digest endosperm. This makes the sugars in these grains more readily available for the body to convert to glucose, causing an insulin spike. Consuming whole grains will still raise blood sugar but at a much more gradual rate. Processed foods are often packed with both refined grains and added sugars. The next section will deal more with nutrition labels so that you can best avoid these refined grains and added sugars in processed foods. There are many resources online for recipes that mimic some processed foods using foods on the lower end of the glycemic index. Cauliflower crust pizza, for example, substitutes the bread crust of a pizza with one made of grated cauliflower, eggs, and cheese. It is not a perfect approximation of a wheat pizza crust but comes without the insulin spike.

How to Interpret Nutrition Labels

Regardless of whether you are choosing to go with a low carb or carb-friendly diet as part of your strategy to reduce insulin resistance and reverse Type 2 Diabetes, learning to decode the nutritional label will help with your diet. Nutritional labels change often and the more recent changes such as labeling the trans fat as well as the added sugar provide even more information that is important when trying to lower insulin resistance. This section will walk through the most important parts of the current nutrition labels used in the United States and how you can use them best.

At the top of the nutrition label are the serving size and servings per container. The serving size can be listed by amount, such as 1/2 cup, but it will also be listed in weight, usually by gram. A common trick food companies use is claiming a smaller serving size so that the calories listed on the table looked smaller. Soda's sold in 20-ounce bottles used to claim a serving size of 8 ounces. When you consume more than the listed serving size, you will have to multiply the other information on the label by the amounts of servings you have eaten.

If you want to be extra precise in determining how many servings you are going to eat, a digital kitchen scale is a good investment. There are several of them on the market for as little as $10. Purchase one with a tare or zeroing function. This enables you to place a bowl on the scale and set the weight to zero before you add the food. To use it with nutrition labels, add the amount you intend to eat and note the amount of grams on the scale. Divide this number by the grams per serving to get the actual amount of servings you are going to eat. This is the number you will need to read the rest of the label.

This might be easier to understand with an example. Let us say that I have a big bag of neon orange cheese puffs. The label states that a serving size is about 21 pieces or 28 grams. I place my snacking bowl on the scale and press the tare or zero button putting the weight back to zero and then add my cheese puffs. The scale reads 78 grams, so to determine how many servings I will be snacking on, I need to divide that number by the number of grams in a serving, 78 / 28 = 3.7, so my snack is actually 3.7 servings and I will have to multiply the information on the label by 3.7 to get an accurate account of what I am about to eat.

The next line of the nutrition label is the amount of calories. Calories represent the potential energy in the food that your body can use to power its cells. As discussed in previous chapters, calories that are not used for energy are stored in the fat for later use, especially simple carbs and sugars. For weight loss, you need to burn more calories than you eat, but for reducing insulin resistance, the amounts of simple carbs and sugars are even more important. Looking at my cheese puffs snack, the calories per serving are 160 but as I poured out 3.7 servings, the calories in my snacking bowl are 592.

As we moved lower into the nutrition labels, it is important to point out one of the fundamentals that these labels are based on, namely the daily caloric intake and corresponding daily value. These are determined based on a 2,000 calorie a day diet which the Food and Drug Administration has determined as the proper intake for an average adult. Your daily diet will vary. The daily values represent the amount of those nutrients the FDA recommends for daily consumption. For battling insulin resistance and reversing Type 2 Diabetes, some of these numbers will be different.

The FDA recommends that 45 to 65 percent of your calories come from carbohydrates while 20 to 35 percent come from fats and 10 to 35 percent come from proteins. Obviously, for those using a low carb diet, the amount of recommended daily carbs will not work with their diet and those who are not limiting their carbs would be better served with a smaller percentage of carbs, especially simple carbs and sugars.

Below the calories per servings, are the listings for fat. This includes separate lines for saturated fats and trans fats. Avoid any foods with trans fats as they have been shown to have several negative health consequences. Saturated fats have been an area of concern over the last seventy years. There is some evidence that they contribute to heart disease but the research in this area is somewhat inconclusive. Some studies show a link while others do not. Low carb dieters often eat larger amounts of saturated fats than recommended with no adverse effect. With my example of cheese puffs, the total fat is 10 grams per serving with 1.5 of them coming from saturated fats and zero trans fat. With my 3.7 serving bowl, I am getting 37 grams of fat with 5.6 of them coming from saturated fats.

Next on the nutrition label is cholesterol. Cholesterol is a waxy substance and in the body it can build up in the arteries, constricting blood flow and ultimately blocking arteries causing strokes. It was long thought that eating foods high in cholesterol such as eggs lead to higher levels of bad cholesterol in the blood so the daily value for cholesterol represents the maximum the FDA recommends and not a goal. Research has changed this view and genetics seems to play a larger role than dietary cholesterol in the level of cholesterol in the blood. If you have a family history of heart disease, limiting cholesterol is likely a good idea. Back to my cheese puff example, there is no cholesterol in them.

Sodium is the next part of the label and like cholesterol, its daily value represents the maximum daily intake. The body requires some sodium, but too much can lead to high blood pressure which can aggravate health issues around insulin resistance and Type 2 Diabetes. So while sodium has no direct effect on blood sugar, reducing your sodium intake should be part of your insulin resistance reversing diet. If you do not have high blood pressure, limit your intake of sodium to the daily value of 2300 mg per day. With the cheese puff example, a serving of cheese puffs has 250 milligrams of sodium, representing 11 percent of the maximum recommended daily intake. With my 3.7 serving bowl that equals 925 mg, just over 40 percent of the maximum recommended daily intake.

Under sodium, we reach the big one for insulin resistance reducing diets, carbohydrates. Like the fat entry, the carbs are broken up into several different lines including fiber, sugars, and added sugars. Fiber plays an important role in slowing the absorption of sugars from digesting carbs but to determine the net carbs, the amount of fiber should be subtracted. Foods that are high in sugar should be avoided but low levels of sugar are fine when the food in question is high in fiber and other carbs unless you are using a low or no carb diet. Added sugars should be avoided completely. These are sugars that are added separately from the other ingredients which make them much easier for the body to digest. The cheese puffs have 15 grams of carbohydrates with less than a gram of fiber and sugar. A good rule of thumb when dealing with 'less than a gram' when determining the amount in your serving is to round positive nutrients down and negative nutrients up. This will better ensure that you do not overindulge. Using that rule, the cheese puffs have 15 grams of net carbs with 1 gram of sugar and no fiber. With my 3.7 serving bowl, that equates to 45 grams of carbs and 3.7 grams of sugar.

The final section of the top half of the nutrition label is protein. This is the only section of the nutrition label that has little controversy or mixed research. Foods high in protein are good for reducing insulin resistance as long as they are not also high in simple carbs and sugars. Looking again at the cheese puff example, there are 2 grams of protein in a serving of cheese puffs so my 3.7 serving bowl will contain 7.4 grams of protein.

The bottom half of the label lists the vitamins and minerals that are present in the food. If you are using a low carb diet, you should be supplementing your diet with vitamin pills or other dietary supplements. This is an advisable strategy for anyone and it makes the lower half of the label generally unimportant.

Reading the ingredient list can be a taxing proposition both due to the small size of the type and the amount of unfamiliar multisyllabic words for the different additives common to processed foods. Some nutritionist advocate avoiding many of these chemicals and there is no reason not to should you desire that, but they generally have little effect on reducing insulin resistance. Refined and enriched flours, on the other hand, should be avoided. These are more simple carbs that will have a greater effect on your blood sugar level.

Chapter 6: Tracking Your Progress

Tracking the success of your insulin resistance reducing diet can be difficult without monitoring your blood sugar levels. Those using a low carb diet have access to tools that can be used to determine if they are in ketoses, but outside of that, the best way to track your success is to document it.

Ketosis Tracking

Ketosis is the state when in starvation or on a very low carb diet when the liver secretes ketone bodies to trigger the cells of the body to convert fatty acids stored in the antipode cells into fuel. A side effect to this is the release of the ketone by-products into the urine and breath. Several products are available to detect these ketone by-products.

Cheapest amongst these products are urine sticks that change colors in the presence of acetoacetic acid in the urine. These are generally pretty easy to use and take under 30 seconds to show if you are in ketosis. On the other hand, some might prefer not to deal with urinating on a strip. Breath ketone monitors are an alternative, though they tend to be more expensive.

There are many models of breath ketone analysis devices on the market. These tend to be electrical and some of them connect with smartphone apps and can be used to track your ketosis over time. While a hundred urine strips can be purchased for $5, breath analysis devices can range in the hundreds of dollars.

A final solution to determine ketosis is blood-based devices. These devices are similar to blood sugar meters and use test strips with drops of blood on them. These machines tend to monitor glucose level as well so they can provide extra information. Again, like the breath monitors, these tend to be expensive.

Tracking Your Diet

Diet tracking has become much easier in the last few years with the rise of smartphones. There is a multitude of different free apps that can be used to track different aspects of your diet from carb and glucose intake to activity level. Specific to diabetes, there are apps that can help you monitor your blood glucose level in addition to other aspects, but even for those who are not testing their blood glucose level, there are apps that will help monitor your diet.

My Fitness Pal is a free calorie counting app that has a database of over 6 million different foods. It can be used to track carbs as well as calories and can also sync with other apps such as Fitbit that track exercise or walking steps. SparkPeople is another calorie and fitness tracking app. Like My Fitness Pal, it is free but also offers a monthly subscription plan with customized workouts and meal plans should you desire. There are dozens of other apps that are available with more being released.

In addition to tracking the progress of your diet with apps, noting your energy levels and mood can also help to track how your level of insulin resistance is lowering. The high blood sugar or hypoglycemia, common to those who suffer from insulin resistance causes fatigue, both physically and mentally, and can lead to mood swings and irritability. By undertaking a diet that removes the sugars and simple carbohydrates that cause blood sugar to be so high, these symptoms will reverse and you will find yourself thinking clearer and having more energy.

By tracking your energy levels and mood, you will be able to monitor any negative changes to your mood. This can be particularly effective to determine the effects of cheating on your diet will have. If you fall off the wagon and overindulge in foods full of sugars and other simple carbs, at the very least, you will notice a drop in energy level the next day. This can also be used when adding different foods to a low carb diet. If you feel that drop in energy the next day or notice an unexplained rise in irritability, cutting back on the added carbs is advisable.

Conclusion

Thank you for reading the Insulin Resistance Diet Plan and we hope that you found it informative. If you put the information provided by this book into practice, you will start to reduce your insulin resistance almost immediately and be on your way to reversing or avoiding Type 2 Diabetes. To get the most out of your new insulin resistance reducing diet, keep at it. Stay away from sugars and other simple carbohydrates. Add some extra activity to your routine to help burn off any glucose your body absorbs from your food to keep your blood sugar down.

Keep track of your progress and monitor your moods and energy levels. When you stop overindulging in sugars and simple carbohydrates, you will notice a boost in energy. Use that to keep motivated and moving on your new diet. A negative feedback loop of too much sugar making your body and mind sluggish leading to obesity and insulin resistance brought you here, use the positive feedback loop that the extra energy your new insulin resistance reducing diet will give you to reverse that.

Everyone stumbles, and you will too. If you fall off the no sugar wagon, don't worry. One of the reasons to monitor your mood and energy levels is to provide yourself with documentation on how quickly they can change based on the type of foods you are eating. You will likely notice the negative effects sugar has on you within hours of cheating. Use this knowledge to stave off later temptations. The power to change your life is within your hands, all you have to do is keep at it.

Immune System:

Boost the Immune System, Heal Your Gut, and Cleanse Your Body Naturally

Introduction

Congratulations on purchasing the *Immune System: Boost the Immune System, Heal Your Gut, and Cleanse Your Body Naturally*, and thank you for doing so. Due to the rising number of health issues that affect people worldwide and the significant increase in autoimmune inflammatory diseases, understanding how your immune system operates has become vital. Autoimmune diseases and digestive issues are more common today than ever before. Having a weak immune system can lead to a wide variety of health problems, ranging from allergic reactions to autoimmune disorders. Our immune system and, in turn, how well it is going to function is greatly affected by what we put into our bodies. It is necessary to eat a wide variety of healthy foods in order for our guts to be healthy and operate as they should. Having a defensive immune system that functions optimally, combined with a healthy gut, can greatly increase health and general well-being. After reading this book, you will better understand how your immune and digestive systems operate and know what you can do to improve them both—including how to eliminate food allergies and sensitivities, reduce stomach bloating, restore good bacteria, and heal a leaky gut.

Many factors of life today—such as high stress levels, too little sleep, eating processed foods, and taking antibiotics—can harm our gut microbiota. If the microbiota of our gut is unbalanced, it affects other parts of our bodies, including our immune system, brain, heart, weight, hormone levels, and the ability to absorb nutrients. The aim of this book is to help readers understand the important link between the immune system and gut health. It is for readers who want to heal their gut microbiota and learn how to cleanse their bodies naturally.

The first chapter of the book will explain what the immune system and gut are and how these two are affected by each other. It is essential to understand this relationship before delving into any other part of the book. Chapter two talks about the wide array of health benefits received from having a defensive immune system along with a healthy gut. These benefits range from increased energy levels, less stress, being able to more easily fight off the common cold, to reduce the risk of certain cancers. Chapter three explains the reasons why some people may have problems associated with their immune system. What may be a surprise to some is that many immune system problems and concerns can be controlled by what foods you decide to put in your body. In chapter four, you will be given checklists, which will help determine whether or not you may have issues with your gut health and immune system. Before setting any goals or beginning your journey towards recovery, you need to take an inventory of your own immune system and gut, listen to your body, and take notes.

Chapters five through eight focus on what you can do to improve your immune system and gut health. Chapter five provides a summary of basic strategies you can use to begin boosting your immune system and improving your gut microbiota. In chapter six, you will learn about healthy dietary habits that can be incorporated into your daily life for better gut health, from foods you should be eating to important lifestyle choices.

Chapter seven focus specifically on foods that can boost your immune system naturally—these foods should make their way onto your shopping list immediately. In chapter eight, you can find specific information on meal planning, which will help you get started on the path to restoring your health. In this chapter, you will also be given a sample seven-day meal plan in order to get ideas for healthy, fun meal planning.

Chapter nine provides an introduction to metabolic disorders and discusses health tips on how to recover from certain ones that are not inherited, specifically metabolic syndrome, also known as Syndrome X. In chapter ten, you will learn about certain eating habits that should be avoided when aiming to improve your immune system and gut health, including specific foods that you should not eat. If you are serious about restoring your gut and boosting your immune system, these foods should immediately be removed from your cupboards and refrigerator. Finally, chapter eleven will provide you with a list of things to look for that will help you determine if your hard work towards gut restoration has been successful. After all, you need to know that it has all been worth your efforts.

There are plenty of books on this subject on the market—thanks again for choosing this one! Every effort was made to ensure it is full of as much useful information as possible. Please enjoy!

Chapter 1: Your Immune System and Gut: What They Are and How They Interact

A deep understanding of your immune system and gut is essential. This chapter will define and examine these two systems in detail. Also, in this chapter, you will have the opportunity to discover how they interact.

The Immune System

Our immune system is crucial for human survival. Without an immune system, parasites, bacteria, and viruses would be free to attack our bodies. Our immune system plays a significant role in keeping us healthy. Spread throughout the body, this complex structure is comprised of a combination of cells, organs, proteins, and tissues working hand-in-hand in defending our bodies against germs and other invaders. When functioning properly, the immune system naturally attacks disease-forming substances that enter the body.

Among the cells that make up this vast network, white blood cells play a particularly important role. White blood cells are stored in the lymphoid organs. The following organs are included in this group:

- Lymph nodes – these small glands are throughout the body and are linked by lymphatic vessels.
- Thymus – situated just below the neck, this gland is between your lungs.
- Bone Marrow – in the center of the bones, this produces red blood cells.
- Spleen – this organ filters your blood and can be found in the upper left portion of the abdomen.

White blood cells come in two basic types: phagocytes, which destroy organisms that invade the body; and lymphocytes, which help the body remember invasive organisms that have previously entered the body, thus aiding in their destruction. Lymphocytes are created in the bone marrow and either stay there (maturing into B cells) or head for the thymus gland (maturing into T cells). Each B cell produces one antibody specifically. For example, one cell might produce an antibody that recognizes the common cold virus, while another produces an antibody against the bacteria that typically cause pneumonia.

A crucial role of the immune system is the ability to recognize our own tissue from foreign tissues. It can do this by discovering proteins that are found on cell surfaces. Our immune system learns to ignore its own proteins early on. It's another story, however, when foreign substances enter the body. When these foreigners (called antigens) enter the body, different cell types work together, recognizing and responding to them. The outcome is unique proteins, called antibodies, which latch themselves onto specific antigens. Short for antibody generator, antigens are any substance that can trigger a response from the immune system. In many cases, they are toxins, fungi, viruses, and bacteria—but in addition to these, it can also be one of your own cells that is dead or malfunctioning. Although antibodies are powerful at noticing what antigens to lock onto, they still need some help in order to destroy them. Here is where the T cells come in, some of which are called "killer cells." When antibodies single out certain invasive antigens, your T cells step up to destroy them while reminding other cells to do their jobs. Antibodies also serve other purposes, such as activating certain proteins that assist in killing infected cells, bacteria, and viruses. This specific set of proteins is also part of the immune system and is called complement. Antibodies stay in our bodies to provide defense for the inevitable time when our immune system comes into contact with that antigen again. A good example here would be the chickenpox. Usually, after having it once, we are unlikely to suffer from it again, as our bodies store a copy of the chickenpox antibody, primed and waiting to destroy the chickenpox when and if it arrives again. This protection is called immunity.

Although everyone's immune system is different, it generally becomes stronger as we get older. This is because as we age, we are exposed to more pathogens (any disease-producing organism) and, in turn, have developed a stronger immunity. You may have noticed that children seem to get sick more often than teenagers and adults —this is because they, being younger, have been exposed to fewer pathogens. Among the three different types of immunity in humans, there are innate (born with), adaptive (acquired throughout life), and passive (borrowed from other sources).

- Innate immunity – All human beings are born with a certain level of immunity towards foreign invaders. The external barrier of our bodies, including our skin and the mucous membranes of the gut and throat, naturally provide our first line of defense against pathogens.

- Adaptive immunity – This is the compilation of different antibodies we acquire through life that we develop to protect us against pathogens we encounter. Our immune system remembers when we are exposed to certain diseases or are vaccinated.

- Passive immunity – This immunity, which is borrowed from another source, lasts only for a short period of time. An example of this is a baby receiving antibodies from the mother through her breast milk. This temporary immunity can protect the baby from certain infections early in life.

After the nervous system, your immune system is the most complex one in the body. We've touched on the various cells, organs, and tissues that comprise it—including the skin, bone marrow, spleen, lymph nodes, and mucous membranes. These all help store or create cells that work constantly to keep your whole body healthy. Another very important factor involved in immune system health is the digestive system. Everything that you put into your body is digested through your gastrointestinal tract, also known as your gut.

The Gut: Your Gastrointestinal Tract

When you hear the word "gut," you may immediately think of your stomach or belly, but in the world of health, it takes on a more complex meaning. The gut refers to the gastrointestinal tract, which pertains to a long tube starting from your mouth to the back passage of your body (anus). As we eat, food first passes through the esophagus, then to the stomach, followed by the small intestine. The small intestine can be divided into three parts: the duodenum, the jejunum, and the ileum. The first one is the duodenum, which is directly connected to the stomach. Curling around the pancreas, it is a tube that is C-shaped. The other two parts, jejunum, and ileum, lay wound at the central abdomen. It is in this body part where everything you eat is assimilated and then absorbed later on into the bloodstream.

Next to ileum is the last part of the small intestine, which is subsequently the foremost portion of your large intestine—caecum. The caecum is then entrenched to the appendix. From here, the large intestine takes a turn upward and takes on a new name, the ascending colon. Then, the intestine takes another turn and crosses the body and is now known as the transverse colon. Afterwards, it takes one more turn downward, and this part is called the descending colon. The final portion of the colon, the sigmoid colon, directs to the rectum, which serves as a temporary storage for stools until they are excreted through the anus.

Now that you have a better image of how exactly food passes through the gastrointestinal tract, we can focus on what the tract as a whole actually does and how it works. Simply put, the gut processes food, from the time it is eaten until it is either passed out as stools or absorbed by the body. The digestive process begins in your mouth. In the mouth, there are salivary glands that release saliva. The chemicals in your saliva, which are called enzymes, work with your teeth to break down food. There are also special chemicals in your saliva that prevent bacteria from causing infections. Now, to move food out of your mouth, you must swallow—and as your muscles contract, food is pushed down through the esophagus. Your tongue is a very strong muscle that aids to push food towards the back of the throat. After passing through the esophagus, your food reaches the stomach, and chemicals that are produced by cells here begin digestion.

Sandwiched by the esophagus and the first part of the small intestine, the stomach is a J-shaped organ, which is about the size of a large sausage when empty. The stomach's primary role is helping you assimilate your food, while the other top priority is storing food until it is ready to be received by the gastrointestinal tract (gut). You are able to eat food and fill your stomach at a much higher rate than how your intestines are able to process it. As this process begins, food is being broken down into basic parts, and only then can it be consumed by the walls of your gut, into the bloodstream, and then delivered around the body. Some liquids and foods are consumed by the stomach lining, although the majority of them are taken by the small intestine. Muscles in your gut walls work to mix food with enzymes that are produced by the body. These muscles are also working hard to transport the food towards the end of your intestinal tract. Indigestible food, along with waste substances and germs, are all passed out of the system as feces.

The process of food digestion is managed by the brain, nervous system, and also by various hormones released by the gut. Before you even take your first bite, your brain sends signals through nerves to your stomach. Your stomach reacts by releasing gastric juices (liquid found in your stomach that is made up of enzymes, acid, and hormones released by glands situated in the inner layers of the stomach wall) that are preparing for the arrival of food. When food reaches the stomach, special receptor cells notice changes and then send their own, new signals.

As food leaves the stomach, it heads for the small intestine. The glands and cells that line the small intestine also produce their own intestinal juice, which aids in digestion—and like the stomach, as the walls contract, food is mixed with these juices to make a smooth transition on to the next part of the tract, the large intestine. This intestine, referred to as the colon, mainly absorbs water, and is wider than the small intestine. Bacteria found in the large intestine aid in the final stages of digestion, and muscle movements here move feces towards the rectum. When stool is existent in the rectum, its walls elongate or widen, again activating special receptor cells. Nerves then serve as a medium of transportation for signals from the receptors to the spinal cord, which subsequently responds by sending the synapses back to the muscles of the rectum, thus upping the back passage's pressure, and this is how you know that you need to go to the toilet.

Immune System-Gut Interaction

Now that you have a better grasp of the functions of your immune and digestive systems, it will be easier to understand how one affects the other. Although many of us don't think of it this way, your gut is a really important barricade between your body and all of the pathogens in the world outside. This is because approximately 70 percent of the cells and tissues that make up your immune system are housed in your gut. This makes your gut a huge player in the immune system. The immune system provides a defense between you and all the dangerous bacteria out there that you might happen to swallow. This is why you don't always get sick from swallowing certain bacteria in your food—for example, when you cook after touching something dirty. The immune system is the main connection between our gut bacteria and how these bacteria influence our health and the possibility of disease. Bacteria live throughout the body, but most of all, it lives in the gut. These bacteria, along with fungi and viruses, exist in unique blends that inhabit various parts of the body. The individual cluster from a specific region of the body is known as microbiota. In this case, we are concerned with gut microbiota, also known as "gut flora." Having a healthy gut depends on a healthy gut microbiota. The combinations of this different microbiota together form your microbiome.

As mentioned above, a large portion of your immune system is in your gastrointestinal tract—therefore, there is a lot of interaction between bacteria in the gut and the body's immune system. For instance, many cells in the gut lining dedicate their lives to releasing large quantities of antibodies into the gut, teaching your immune system how to behave. The bacteria in your gut also help maintain a balanced immune system. Having a diverse gut flora teaches the cells of your immune system that not everything it comes into contact with is necessarily bad. This recognition is developed throughout life, as our gut is constantly exposed to new things through food and what we encounter in our surroundings. Due to the fact that the balance of our gut microbiota influences our immune system balance, an unbalanced gut flora can shift the immune system to an inflammatory state, known as "leaky gut."

Chapter 2: The Benefits of a Healthy Gut Combined with a Strong Immune System

No one likes getting sick. We ask ourselves, how do we avoid the latest "bug" that is going around? How can we ensure that every member of our family won't be laid up and feeling low? The answer: a healthy immune system. As we learned in chapter one, a healthy gut promotes a healthy immune system. As your immune system is your body's natural defense system, it is vital to your health that you ensure that it is working properly. The bacteria in your gut support the immune system in a number of ways. Having a strong immune system allows us to fight off infection quickly. The common cold should not last more than a week or so, but for an unhealthy person with a jeopardized natural defense mechanism, it may hang around much longer—or seven come back again and again. The ability to quickly fight off infection isn't the only benefit of a strong immune system-healthy gut combo. Other benefits include boosted energy levels, improved mental health, improved cholesterol levels, regulated hormone levels, less weight gain, a longer life, and better overall health and general well-being.

Boosted Energy levels

We all would like to have more energy, right? Often times you might say to yourself, "If I only had the energy…but I'm so tired!" A good way to start increasing your energy levels is by eating healthy, nutritious foods, but without a healthy gut, your body cannot as easily absorb nutrients from the foods you take in. If you maintain a healthy gut, the body can absorb more nutrients, in turn increasing your energy levels.

Improved Mental Health

Researchers have found that restoring an unhealthy gut can lead to improved mental health. There is definitely a connection between your gut and your mood. If you have ever used the phrase "butterflies in my stomach," then you have proven that this is true. Within our bodies we actually have a so-called second brain, called the enteric nervous system (ENS). This system regulates and controls our intestinal tract and senses threats from the environment. The ENS sends information to the brain through the vagus nerve, which links a number of organs with the brain. About 90 percent of the signals passing along this nerve are traveling from the gut to the brain. This is why it should not be surprising that more than half of those suffering from irritable bowel syndrome (IBS) also suffer from mood disorders, and a common pharmaceutical treatment given for this syndrome is antidepressants. In turn, it has recently been discovered that mood disorders can also be treated from the bottom up, so to speak. In other words, conditions such as depression, anxiety, and sleeping disorders can be effectively treated by restoring the good bacteria in your gut. Many of the psychological problems we are experiencing today may be attributed to what we put into our bodies and how this affects gut flora. Our health can suffer when anything gets in the way of the communication between our gut and our brain.

Better Cholesterol Levels

Good gut bacteria can also improve cholesterol levels. Much of the cholesterol produced by the liver gets converted into bile acids. These are stored in the gallbladder and are then used to aid in digesting fats. These acids then end up in the colon, and here they are either destroyed or leave the body through bowel movements. Those of us who don't eat enough fiber often have a higher amount of disease-causing flora in their gut, leading to an accumulation of cholesterol in the bloodstream. This causes cholesterol level to rise. Also, less cholesterol is able to reach the colon where it can then be let out of the body. This can be very dangerous, as bowel movements are the body's main way of getting rid of unwanted cholesterol. It is essential to eat a high-fiber diet, as this allows your body to get rid of more unwanted cholesterol.

Regulated Hormone Levels

Having a strong immune system and healthy gut microbiota can also regulate hormone levels. Usually, up to 60 percent of the estrogen circulating in the blood is picked up by the liver and then essentially dumped into the gallbladder. It is then released, with bile, into the intestines for excretion. In the gastrointestinal tract, our good gut bacteria produce an enzyme which reactivates the estrogen in order for it to be reabsorbed by the body. When our gut flora is not in balance, the estrogen is neither reabsorbed nor reactivated and instead gets lost in the stool. When women have low estrogen levels, they have a higher risk of osteoporosis, water retention, severe menstrual cramps, PMS, heavy flow and migraine headaches. A similar process happens with other hormones, as well as vitamin B12, vitamin D, cholesterol, folic acid, and bile acids.

Prevents Unhealthy Weight Gain

A healthy gut prevents unhealthy weight (or fat) gain. Restoring the good bacteria in your gut prevents overeating, which leads to gaining weight. There is a lot of research coming out that directly connects our weight with the health, including the amount and type, of our gut flora. When you are carrying extra weight, you face a much higher than average risk of developing many health problems. These conditions include the nation's leading causes of death, such as certain cancers, heart disease, stroke, and diabetes. It should also be noted that carrying around extra weight can also lead to depression.

Longer Lifespan

The healthy immune system-healthy gut combination also contributes to a longer life. When we have more diverse bacterial flora, it becomes more effective, and in turn, our overall health tends to be better. In order to have more diverse bacteria, it is necessary to have a varied diet. This is key to maintaining healthy gut flora, and in the long run, strength and vitality.

Chapter 3: The Causes of Immune System Problems

Many people have problems related to the health of their immune system and gut. Over the past 100 years, our diet has changed dramatically due to the industrialization of our food supply. This modern diet consisting of highly processed, high-fat, high-sugar, and low-fiber foods has greatly altered the bacteria in our gut. Generations ago, these types of foods were not as readily available as they are today, if at all.

The Modern Diet

The food we decide to put into our bodies feeds our fat cells and also determines what kind of garden, or flora, we are growing in our insides. The personal garden inside our gut is filled with bugs that decide more about your mental and emotional well-being that you could imagine. Simply put, if your gut bacteria are sick, so are you. Your gut bacteria thrive on what you feed them, so keep them healthy! You might not correlate digestive issues with allergies, mood disorders, arthritis and certain autoimmune diseases including irritable bowel syndrome and chronic fatigue, however many ailments that do not seem to be related are actually caused by problems in your gut garden. When there are too many bad gut bugs present, or not enough good ones, problems arise that can seriously affect your health and weight. Studies have also shown that people who suffer from obesity and have lower levels of healthy bacteria in the gut continue to gain more weight over time.

There are many reasons why your digestive system may be off balance, leading to a weakened immune system, and an unhealthy diet is the biggest culprit. A diet low in nutrients can damage our inner garden, as it promotes the growth of the bad kind of bacteria.

Stress

Stress is another contributing factor to an unbalanced digestive system. Chronic stress can alter the nervous system in your gut, causing it to leak, while changing its normal bacteria. Other elements that can imbalance your digestive system include medication overuse (including anti-inflammatories and antibiotics), inadequate digestive enzymes, a toxin overload, and infections. The immune system's overall vitality is highly dependent on the person's stress level, emotional stability, nutritional status, dietary practices, and lifestyle.

Genetics

Some people inherited specific genes that make them reactive to elements in their surroundings, which would have otherwise been normal. These matters are referred to as allergens. The most common example of an overactive immune system is to have an allergic reaction. Pollen, mold, dust and some foods are examples of allergens. Some conditions caused by an overactive immune system include eczema (an itchy rash known as atopic dermatitis), asthma (reaction of your lungs that can induce trouble breathing, coughing, or wheezing), and allergic rhinitis (a swelling of the nasal passages along with sneezing and runny nose).

In certain autoimmune diseases, the body attacks what is normal, healthy tissue. A common autoimmune disease is Type 1 diabetes. Here, the immune system attacks cells in the pancreas, which are tasked to create insulin. Insulin then eliminates sugar from the blood in order to utilize it as energy. Another common autoimmune problem is rheumatoid arthritis. In this type of arthritis, the joints begin to swell and become deformed. Lupus is another autoimmune disease that attacks body tissues, such as the lungs, skin, and kidneys.

Serious immune system disorders are just some of the possible outcomes of a faulty immune system. A person with an immune system disorder may:

- Have an immune system that has turned against itself. This is called an autoimmune disease.
- Inherit a weak immune system. This is called primary immune deficiency.
- Develop an ailment that weakens the immune system. This is called acquired immune deficiency.
- Have an immune system that is overactive. This causes an allergic reaction.
- Have a cancer of the immune system.

Common examples of immune system disorders include:

- Temporary acquired immune deficiencies. This is when your immune system is temporarily deteriorated by something, such as a medicine. This may happen to chemotherapy patients due to the medications utilized to fight cancer. Additionally, it affects those who have recently had organ transplants and that are taking medicine to prevent rejection of the organ. Furthermore, infections like the flu virus, measles, and mononucleosis can dwindle your immune system within a short period of time. Poor nutrition, drinking alcohol in excess and smoking can all also lead to a temporarily weakened immune system.

- Severe combined immunodeficiency (SCID). This immune deficiency is present at birth, as children born with it are missing important white blood cells.

- Acquired Immune Deficiency Syndrome (AIDS). Human Immunodeficiency Virus (HIV), which causes AIDS, is a viral infection which destroys white blood cells and weakens the immune system. People affected become seriously ill with infections that other people can fight off.

Chapter 4: Take Stock of Your Gut Health and Immune System

Do you wonder if your gut is unhealthy—or if your immune system is weak? Does your gut or immune system need help or support? Maybe yes, maybe no. Paying close attention to your body is one of the greatest things you can do for yourself and is the first step in answering these questions. Taking an inventory of how you are feeling and taking note of anything that seems off is also a good way to start. Knowing the signs of a weak immune system is important because these are red flags that allow you the chance to resolve health problems before they become more serious.

Your Gut

Let's start with our gut. Our intestines are permeable, meaning they allow the good nutrients we receive through the food we eat to pass into the bloodstream and nourish us. The intestines also function to keep bad microbes and toxins in the gut temporarily to eventually be passed out as waste. However, when we feed our intestines the wrong types of foods and treat them with inactivity and stress, they cannot function properly. Sometimes, these toxins and microbes escape the gut and are released into the bloodstream, causing inflammation and leading to what is known as "leaky gut." The leaky gut syndrome is not a legitimate medical term but is the name given to describe damage to the lining of your intestines, allowing proteins that are not digested to enter your bloodstream. It is also called "increased intestinal permeability." Below is a list of symptoms associated with the leaky gut syndrome.

- Stomach bloating, gas, constipation, diarrhea or irritable bowel syndrome
- Chronic fatigue or fibromyalgia (constant pain that is spread throughout the body, typically lasting more than three months)

- Frequent colds
- Depression, anxiety, ADHD
- Unhealthy weight
- Joint pain
- Headaches
- Food allergies or sensitivities
- Thyroid conditions
- Autoimmunity
- Rosacea, eczema, acne or psoriasis
- Hormonal imbalances
- Autoimmune disorders such as rheumatoid arthritis, Hashimoto's thyroiditis, lupus, psoriasis or celiac disease

If you have several of these symptoms, it is time to start restoring your unhealthy gut.

Another common gastrointestinal problem is irritable bowel syndrome. Do you consider your digestive tract to be irritable? There are an estimated 10 to 15 percent of people suffering from irritable bowel syndrome around the world, and of that percentage, somewhere between 25 and 45 million are living in the United States. Signs of irritable bowel syndrome vary greatly, but can include:

- Constipation
- Diarrhea
- Hard, dry stools one day and watery the next
- Bloating
- Feeling the need to rush to the bathroom

As with many other ailments of the gut, treatment centers largely on diet, avoiding triggers such as alcohol and caffeine and trying to reduce stress.

While not nearly as common as irritable bowel syndrome, celiac disease is also worth mentioning here, as it is an autoimmune and digestive disorder. Only about one percent of the U.S. population has a celiac disease diagnosis, and its sufferers are unable to consume gluten. Gluten is a protein mainly found in wheat, rye, and barley. When people with celiac disease eat gluten, an attack is triggered on their small intestine. It should be noted that only about five percent of people with celiac disease actually get diagnosed as having it. This leaves close to approximately three million Americans suffering from its symptoms without even knowing they have the disease. Apart from this population, there is another 15-20 percent of Americans living with a gluten sensitivity.

Symptoms of celiac disease vary, but can include:

- Chronic diarrhea
- Abdominal bloating and pain
- Vomiting
- Constipation
- Pale or fatty stool

Celiac disease is diagnosed with stool samples and blood tests. There is no cure for it, and sufferers must adopt a gluten-free diet, and accidentally eating a product containing gluten can cause an immediate flare-up.

Your Immune System

Now that a few checklists have been provided in order to take an inventory of your gut, we cannot forget about the immune system, as there are many signs indicating you may have one that is weak. Below is a list of questions that you can ask yourself to determine whether or not yours is up to par.

1. Do I have persistent colds?

On average, the common cold lasts seven to ten days. The immune system can take up to three or four days to develop antibodies to fight it off. If you have a cold that lasts longer than ten days, your immunity might be struggling.

2. At times are my lymph glands sore and swollen?

These bean-shaped glands are especially easy to find in your neck, armpits, and groin, and swell up when they are fighting off injury or infection. If persistent swelling occurs, this might mean that your immune system is having a difficult time fighting off a problem.

3. Do I catch colds easily?

4. Do I suffer from repeated infections?

We all develop infections now and then, after all, we are only human. But when your immune system is weak, it has a much harder time killing pathogens. The result is infections that return over and over.

5. Do I constantly feel fatigued?

If your immune system is struggling, so does your level of energy. This is because your body is trying to conserve this energy to power your immune system. As a result, you will feel tired. This can be frustrating when you are trying to work, and get the many things accomplished that you need to throughout your day. Fatigue is worth paying attention to when it becomes persistent.

6. Do I have wounds that take a really long time to heal?

Your skin enters into a state of damage control when you get a burn, cut or scrape. Our bodies work to protect the wound by bringing nutrient-rich blood to the area so it can regenerate new skin. This necessary process of wound healing is highly dependent on healthy immune cells. When your immune system is weak, however, your skin will find it difficult to regenerate, and the wound would refuse to heal.

In case any of those previous questions got you to agree, it is a signal that your immune system may need support, and this support can come in the form of taking measures to heal your gut. Chronic or recurrent infections, even mild colds, only occur when one has a weakened immune system. Under these circumstances, there is a cycle that repeats itself: a deteriorated immune system directs to the infection, and infection then induces harm to the immune system, which consequently abates the body's resistance even further. However, improving the immune system through better gut health can break this vicious cycle.

Chapter 5: Improving Your Immune System and Gaining a Healthier Gut

After making it through the first four chapters, you now have a better understanding of how the immune system and gastrointestinal tract work together. You know the benefits to your health and well-being when they are functioning optimally. You understand immune system problems and the reasons why they make people suffer. Also, you have taken an inventory of your own gut and immune system. Now, you are ready to learn about ways you can boost your immune system and restore an unhealthy gut. Your gut health literally affects the whole body, so if you want to fix your health, you need to start with your gut. Your gut is constantly at work performing many important jobs, including breaking down food, keeping out toxins, and producing and absorbing nutrients. If optimal immunity is what you desire, your gut must function flawlessly.

As more than 100 million Americans suffer from digestive problems, much research has been done on how to strengthen your intestinal lining and improve digestion. You are definitely not alone if you suffer from, or have suffered from, a digestive disorder, such as stomach bloating, constipation, irritable bowel syndrome, gas, diarrhea, heartburn or acid reflux. Out of the five best-selling drugs in the U.S., two are for digestive problems, and they cost billions of dollars. Furthermore, there are more than 200 over-the-counter drugs out there for digestive disorders, and most of these can cause further digestive ailments. Trips to the doctor for intestinal disorders are very common, and many of us do not realize that problems in the gut affect the entire body, leading to a wide array of concerns, including allergies, autoimmune disease, arthritis, acne, mood disorders, fatigue and more. Your gut's health defines what nutrients can be consumed, and what microbes are to be expelled. Essentially, it's directly responsible for your body's overall health.

You need to begin by focusing on improving your gut microbiota. Your body contains trillions of microbes, and the densest population is in your gut. Here they play a critical role in immune function, weight regulation and digestion. What you eat can quickly alter the balance of your gut microbiota. Before talking more about what you can do to improve your microbiome overall, here are a few facts about microbes.

- The bacteria in our gut can weigh over four pounds.
- Analysis of gut bacteria can predict obesity with a 90% accuracy rate.
- Our bodies contain 100 trillion microbes.
- Less than five percent of microbes actually cause disease.
- There are more microbes on your hand that there are people on the planet.
- Bacteria influences our behavior through neurons in our gut, that is why our gut is considered to be our second brain.
- Studies have associated a healthy microbial balance with lower incidences of heart disease, diabetes, cancer, asthma, depression, liver disease, autism, irritable bowel syndrome, colic, and many allergies.

Your Gut Microbiota

Your gut microbiota changes with every bite of food you take, so the good news is that you have the power to restore good bacteria in your gut immediately. What you eat isn't just for you, it is also nourishing the trillions of bacteria living in your gut. You can positively change your gut flora starting with your very next meal. You need to feed your gut bacteria the right food and fertilize your personal inner gut garden. If you feed them fresh, whole, real foods, you will have a happy, healthy gut. On the other hand, if you feed them junk, the bad bugs will flourish, resulting in leaky gut and inflammation. Certain fat-regulating hormones then get out of whack, and you end up craving more bad foods. Over time, however, as you continue to eat healthily, these cravings will decrease. Once you start to notice a difference in the way you feel, you may not even desire the less healthy foods that once filled your cupboards and refrigerator, because you know how bad you can feel when your bacteria are unbalanced by junk food and sugar.

Cultivating and Restoring a Healthy Gut

We already know about this complex collection of bacteria living in our gastrointestinal tract, our unique gut microbiota, but now it is time to find out more about the control we have over how it makes us feel. The following are ways you can cultivate, as well as restore, good bacteria in your gut.

Increase dietary fiber intake.

Changing your diet is the most direct and best way to go about transforming your gut flora. Eating more plants allows us to achieve and maintain diversity in our microbiota. This diversity will lead to a clearer mind and a better mood. Similar to how sugar is processed too easily and in turn starves our gut flora, dietary fiber gives our microbiota plenty to feast on, highly benefiting our internal garden. Eating foods that are high in dietary fiber will keep your intestinal lining intact, and will also help maintain a more diverse collection of good bacteria, vital to good health.

Limit antibiotic use.

At certain points in our lives, antibiotic use is unavoidable. Regular antibiotic use, however, kills our diverse mini-ecosystem of microbiota and poses more health hazards. Broad types of antibiotics don't differentiate between what is beneficial for our health and what is harmful, sometimes damaging certain strains of bacteria that we need to fight other infections.

Take probiotics.

The use of a probiotic supplement can also be beneficial when aiming to restore an unhealthy gut. Probiotics are certain foods or supplements that contain living microbes. These microbes when ingested are intended to improve and support your microbiome's health, strengthening or replacing the communities of bacteria currently in the gut.

Probiotics vs. Prebiotics

To avoid confusion, a note should be added here about the difference between prebiotics and probiotics. Prebiotics are foods that sort of fertilize the bacteria already existing in our gut and encourage the development of diversity. These foods are complex carbohydrates, such as whole grains and vegetables. As mentioned above, probiotics are foods that contain live bacteria thought to be beneficial to the body.

Actively reduce stress.

When you are feeling stressed, your body naturally releases adrenaline, and your immune system discharges inflammatory proteins that are important in cell signaling, called cytokines. This happens regardless of whether or not whatever you are feeling stressed about is real or not. For example, a possible attack by a wild animal versus worrying about the presentation you have to give at work tomorrow. If you are feeling stressed all the time, your immune response never stops sending these inflammation messages all over your body, including to the bugs in your gut, weakening its health and causing inflammation. For the sake of our guts and our immune system, we really need to try to chill out.

Get sufficient sleep.

We can balance our gut flora by consistently getting enough sleep, as close to eight hours as possible being the recommendation. The relationship between our microbiome and sleep is looked at as a two-way street. The microbiota in our gut has an effect of how we sleep, and sleep also appears to affect the diversity and health of our gut garden. Not getting enough sleep decreases types of beneficial bacteria in the gut and can quickly cause negative effects on the microbiome and immune health.

Exercise regularly.

Our gut microbiota loathes a sedentary body and is much happier when we exercise. It has been shown that exercise actually induces a different type of change in our gut flora than a diet, for example. Exercise changes the composition of your gut microbiota, and studies have shown that these positive changes can occur after only six weeks of exercising. It is important to point out that the exercise must be continued regularly to continue to notice these changes, otherwise regression will occur. Even moderate exercise can improve cholesterol levels. Although, regular exercise, 30 minutes a day five days a week, helps ward off metabolic syndrome. Exercise is a key component in boosting your metabolism and keeping your weight down.

Drink more water.

When you drink more water and stay hydrated, your gut microbiota is happy and healthy, allowing it to fully support other parts of your body. There are different opinions on how much water you should drink every day, but it is commonly recommended to drink eight 8-ounce glasses, which is equal to about 2 liters or have a gallon. Referred to like the 8x8 rule, it is easy to remember. Drinking enough water throughout the day can seem like a chore to some, and if you are one of these people, try using some kind of fun container or glass that you love, one that makes you smile when you use it. It sure is more fun than chugging from the same boring cup, and it also sets you up for success from a psychological standpoint. The pleasure you receive from using the container is seen as a reward by your brain, and it triggers a release of dopamine. This makes you more likely to want to keep performing the action that leads to the reward, it this case the reward is drinking out of the fun container. You end up consuming more water, benefiting your gut.

Having your digestion recover will take some time, but know that doing so is possible. If you want vibrant health, you must focus on your gut first. There are many things that you can do to improve your immune system and have a healthier gut, and following the recommendations above is a great place to start. Keep these in mind as you begin the healing process, and watch your symptoms decline, and eventually disappear.

Chapter 6: Heal Your Gut With Healthy Diets

As mentioned throughout this book so far, the foods we eat greatly impact our gut health and immune system. There are many healthy diet plans that we can follow and other things that we can do to put ourselves on the right path towards better health and well-being. Whether you want to reduce stomach bloating, eliminate food allergies, or boost your immune system, it all starts in the gut. An important thing to remember is that what contributes to a healthy gut is the consumption of real, fresh, whole foods.

Rebalancing Your Gut

The foundation of great gut health starts with what you eat. Your focus should be on fiber-rich vegetables, non-gluten grains, low-sugar fruits, and legumes. The immune system boosting and gut healing process in many cases follow these steps:

1. Remove the bad bacteria and food allergens in the gut that are causing sensitivities. This can be done by eliminating inflammatory foods such as soy, corn, gluten, dairy, sugar, and eggs. Other irritants such as caffeine and alcohol should also be avoided.

2. Replace the bad bacteria through healthy food choices that contain needed enzymes, fiber, and prebiotics.

3. Restore a healthy balance of bacteria by introducing new, beneficial bacteria, maybe through a probiotic supplement.

4. Repair the lining of your gut with healing nutrients such as omega 3 fatty acids.

Below are some healthy dietary measures that should be taken when you are trying to heal your gut.

Eliminate certain food.

Sometimes, a food elimination diet may be in order to address food sensitivities in the body. When it comes to gut health, there are some foods that should be avoided for the long haul if possible. Processed foods, gluten, and soy top the list as main offenders that should be eliminated. All three of these are harmful to the gut lining. Processed foods are far from real, containing sugars, oils, and additives. As modern soy and gluten are often genetically modified, they also can contribute to tearing up our gut lining. Eliminating certain other foods, such as dairy, yeast, corn, and eggs for a week or two is also recommended. After the elimination, see how your gut feels and notice changes in other symptoms you may have been experiencing. Sometimes you can gradually re-introduce these foods or replace them with more gut-friendly options.

Eat a wide variety of foods.

As our bodies were not meant to eat the same foods every day, it is important for gut health to vary the foods that you are eating. In the past, the easy access to all different types of foods throughout the entire year that we experience today was not possible. Living in a northern climate, for example, one could not go to the grocery store and find mangos and kiwis in the winter. People back then ate seasonally. What was growing around them during a specific season was what they ate. If you want to restore healthy bacteria in your gut, you must eat a wide variety of foods to allow your gut flora to diversify and grow. Try paying more attention to what is in season, choosing fresh foods that don't have to travel too far to get to your plate. Aim to rotate the foods you eat more often, for example, if you eat lots of broccoli on Monday, try not to eat it again until Friday, choosing other seasonal vegetables the days in between. Also, eating a variety of different foods keeps things interesting and makes meal planning more enjoyable.

Don't gulp down water with meals.

Of course, it is beneficial to drink lots of water throughout the day. However, drinking large amounts of water during meals can dilute the digestive juices that are hard at work digesting what you are feeding your gut, sometimes interfering with the process as a whole. During meals, take small sips of water, and drink the majority of your water between meals.

Eat in a relaxed state.

This is by far one of the most important pieces of healing an unhealthy gut. Feeling stressed or rushed while eating impairs digestion. If you are eating while driving through heavy traffic or trying to have breakfast while rushing out the door in the morning, your body is not in a relaxed state. A conscious effort must be made to put your body in a relaxed state before eating, and you might need to make adjustments in your daily schedule so that you are able to fully enjoy meal time. Try turning off your phone before dinner, and focus on what you are eating and how it is nourishing your body. Try to allow at least 20-30 minutes for meals, as this is how long it takes our stomach to signal to the brain that it is feeling satisfied or full. If you can, allow your food some time to settle before leaving the table. When we eat too fast, we can sometimes end up eating more food than we need to before realizing that we are full.

Chapter 7: Foods That Naturally Boost Immune System

Learning how to boost your immune system through what you put in your gut is the next step on the journey toward cleansing your body naturally. When people are trying to improve their immune system, they hear about many treatments out there that claim to be cure-all remedies, promising to boost immunity and lessen chances of getting colds and flu. These remedies may be over-the-counter medications, the flu shot, or supplements. Although these can possibly offer preventative benefits, the real key to boosting immunity is lesser-known: cultivating healthy, diverse bacteria in the gut. Food should be looked at as medicine for your body, which can naturally give you a stronger immunity. What follows is a list of easily acquired foods that will aid in your goal of a having and maintaining a healthy gut.

Fiber-Rich Produce

It will be necessary to increase your intake of fruits and vegetables, especially those that are rich in prebiotic fiber. Dietary prebiotics is non-digestible compounds of fiber that pass undigested through the upper portion of your gut and encourage the growth of good bacteria. Fruits and veggies high in prebiotic fiber include bananas, onions, garlic, mushrooms, chicory, asparagus, and Jerusalem artichokes. You will also want to eat plenty of other colorful, nourishing vegetables like broccoli, cabbage, cauliflower, Brussel's sprouts, sweet potatoes, bok choy, and leafy greens.

Having a fiber deficiency can lead to various health problems, so it is essential to get enough of this important nutrient. Fiber is one of the most crucial ingredients for gut health, and only about three percent of Americans are ingesting the recommended 40 grams of fiber they need every day. Fiber feeds the good bacteria in our gut, promoting the health of your microbiome and boosting your immune system. Our gut microbiota extract fiber's vitamins, nutrients and energy, decreasing inflammation and protecting against obesity. There are two types of fiber. Soluble fiber helps lower cholesterol and can be found in oatmeal, legumes (peas, beans, nuts, and lentils) and some fruits and vegetables. Insoluble fiber gives your digestive environment a more cleansing effect and can be found in whole grains, kidney beans, and fruits and veggies too.

Bananas and Apples

One of the most popular foods in the world, bananas are extremely good at restoring harmony in your gut microbiota. They contain potassium and magnesium, which assists in the prevention of inflammation. It has been proven that bananas reduce stomach bloating and help your body to release excess weight. There are many easy ways to incorporate more bananas into your diet, such as in smoothies, sliced on top of cereal or simply as an afternoon snack.

Like bananas, apples are easy to find, high in fiber and boost the good bacteria in your gut. Apples can be enjoyed raw as a snack or stewed.

Cultured or Fermented Foods

Cultured and fermented foods are rich in probiotics that promote diversity in your gut leading to a strengthened immune system. The shelf life of fermented foods is prolonged through an old-fashioned process, which subsequently increases its nutritional value. They also provide live, healthy microorganisms and probiotics to your body. The foods that give you these healthy probiotics are fermented using a natural process which actually contains probiotics. If you are unsure whether or not the foods you are choosing contain these healthy probiotics, the label should contain the words "naturally fermented." Examples of these foods include yogurt, kimchi, kefir, sauerkraut, apple cider vinegar, and kombucha tea, among others. In the past, there used to be more priority placed on consuming fermented foods than there is now, which may be contributing to less diversity in gut microbiota today.

Bone Broths

Bone broths such as beef, chicken, turkey, and fish are rich in gut healing nutrients. They have long been a staple in the diet of humans, but homemade broths are not as popular as they used to be due to how easy it now is to purchase store-bought stocks. However, what is gaining in popularity is the use of bone broths as a healing agent in gut health. To make bone broth, you cook meat or fish in water, usually with vegetables, for an extended period of time. Cooking times vary widely, from three hours to as many as 72 hours. It is better to make your own broth than to use store-bought, as this way you know exactly what is in it. Store-bought broths can also be processed, stripping it of its natural healing properties.

Omega-3 Fatty Acids

Omega-3 fatty acids regulate the passage of nutrients and waste products in your body and also promote healthy signaling between cells. Many studies have found that by increasing your intake of omega-3's you can increase microbe diversity in your gut. These acids also maintain the very important upkeep of your intestinal wall. We cannot make these essential fatty acids in our body, so we must get them from our food. Oily fish including salmon, mackerel, sardines, anchovies, oysters, caviar and herring contain a high amount of omega-3 fatty acids. Other animal products including grass-fed and organic lamb, elk, chicken, bison, goat, beef, rabbit and pasture-raised eggs are also good sources of omega 3's. You can also get omega– 3's from other foods such as flaxseed, walnuts and chia seeds, although in smaller amounts. Flaxseed contains insoluble fiber and helps improve regularity in your digestive tract. It also has the highest content of lignans (antioxidants carrying anti-cancer properties) of any food out there. Like other foods covered in this chapter, flaxseed promotes good gut flora. After grinding the seed, it can be used in smoothies, sprinkled on salads or added to recipes when baking. Remember to keep your flaxseed in the freezer, as it can go rancid quickly.

Wild-caught fish and offal

Organ meats such as liver, found from high-quality sources, are full of nutrients and healthy fats, and the same goes for wild caught fish. If you eat these often, you are giving your body what it needs to heal.

Polyphenols

Polyphenols are plant compounds that offer many benefits to your health. A few of these benefits include a reduction in cholesterol levels, blood pressure, and inflammation. Some sources of polyphenols include almonds, blueberries, onions, broccoli, grape skins, red wine, cocoa, and dark chocolate. Polyphenols can't always be digested by human cells, but they are efficiently broken down by the microbiota in our gut.

Take healthy fats.

Fats are needed by the body to help control inflammation. Healthy fats include olives and unrefined olive oil, avocado and unrefined avocado oil, coconut and unrefined coconut oil, butter from grass-fed cows and high-quality animal fats. Poor quality fats such as certain seed oils produce more inflammation.

Add these foods to your shopping list today!

Chapter 8: Plan Meals to Restore Your Health

Planning your meals should be fun, not a chore. As we gain a better understanding of and take more interest in what happens to our overall health and well-being by nourishing our bodies with healthy foods, the more enjoyable meal planning becomes. It may be difficult at first to know how to plan meals around gut-healthy foods, and this chapter's aim is to give you examples of meals that you can plan to be used for gut restoration. A healthy gut menu should always be centered on vegetables, fruits, and lean protein. Cultured dairy products and fermented vegetables are excellent additions because they offer a great supply of healthy gut bacteria.

Focus on Food Preparation

Sometimes, the way a food is prepared can change the way it affects the body. For example, fried meats are very different that slow-cooked meats. You should focus on meats that are slow cooked or cooked at low temperatures, vegetables that are very well cooked and seeds and nuts that are soaked and sprouted. Foods prepared this way are easier on our digestive system, and the nutrients are also easier to absorb. Again, after your unhealthy gut becomes healthy, you can slowly reintroduce foods cooked in other ways, and see how your body responds.

Another good rule is to only eat junk food that you have cooked yourself. Making your own "junk food" from scratch helps you cut out a lot of the harmful ingredients found in processed snacks and fast foods, such as artificial flavors and colors, emulsifiers, preservatives, and hydrogenated fats and oils. All of these ingredients harm your gut. When you begin to prepare everything you eat yourself, you will become more mindful of the foods you eat and your palette will become more sensitive.

Balance your meals.

It is important to balance the nutrient ratios of what you have on your plate. If you don't, sometimes you can spike your blood sugar with too many carbohydrates, or make it drop by eating too little fat or protein. Having a proper balance is necessary for proper digestion and feeling full. You don't want to eat a whole meal and then feel hungry after only an hour. This leads to overeating and weight gain. Balancing your meals is an ongoing process, and there is no one-size-fits-all strategy. However, you can start by filling your plate with 30% protein, 30% fat and 40% vegetables. Then listen to your body and take an inventory, noticing how your digestion feels after you eat, and how hungry you are between meals. Remember that a healthy plate of food will feature several different colors. The colors of many different vegetables reflect the different phytochemicals and antioxidants that they contain, all of which are aiding to reduce inflammation and feed our gut bacteria.

Start Your Own Vegetable Garden

Starting your own vegetable garden can have many benefits. The soil is rich in microbes and gardening is a rewarding activity. Just knowing that you grew the vegetables that you are eating provides a lot of personal satisfaction. Also, your grocery bill is likely to decrease when you stop buying produce from the grocery store. The uncertainty of whether or not your vegetables have been sprayed with harmful pesticides will also not be a concern.

Here is a sample meal plan for one week. These are suggestions only, as you are now more aware of what kind of foods you should have in your diet, you can play around a bit and make new and interesting food combinations.

Sample Meal Plan

Day 1

Breakfast: Pineapple, kale and almond milk smoothie
Lunch: Brown rice salad with kale, spinach, carrots, and beets
Dinner: Baked chicken, with beans, roasted carrots, and broccoli

Day 2

Breakfast: Zucchini frittata with mushroom and spinach
Lunch: Stuffed sweet potato halves, filled with turkey, cranberries, and spinach
Dinner: Grilled chicken wings with sauerkraut and fresh spinach on the side

Day 3

Breakfast: Chia pudding with coconut and papaya. One cup unsweetened coconut milk, a quarter cup of chia seeds and a quarter cup of diced papaya
Lunch: Chicken salad, with an olive oil dressing
Dinner: Roasted tempeh with broccoli over brown rice

Day 4

Breakfast: Oatmeal, gluten-free, topped with a quarter cup of raspberries
Lunch: Leftovers from the previous night's dinner
Dinner: Steak with sweet potatoes and Brussel's sprouts

Day 5

Breakfast: Greek yogurt, banana, and blueberry smoothie

Lunch: Salad of mixed greens with sliced hard-boiled eggs
Dinner: Stir-fried beef and broccoli with sauerkraut over noodles

Day 6

Breakfast: Omelet with your choice of veggies.
Lunch: Egg frittata with salmon and veggies
Dinner: Grilled chicken salad with sauerkraut on the side

Day 7

Breakfast: Greek yogurt smoothie with blueberry and almond milk (unsweetened)
Lunch: Leftovers from the previous night's dinner
Dinner: Grilled salmon over a fresh garden salad

Bonus: A Recipe for Bone Broth

It is also beneficial, as mentioned earlier, to consume a homemade bone broth. Bone broth not only repairs your gut lining but also contains glutamine, a fuel for cells in your intestine that might help your leaky gut. Drinking a cup of bone broth each day can also help when you are managing heavy stress or are running low on sleep. You can buy bones from a local butcher to make homemade broth. If making beef broth, aim to source beef marrow bones from certified grass-fed cows. The following outlines steps for making a homemade beef bone broth.

Step 1

Put about two and a half pounds of beef marrow bones and two and a half pounds of beef soup bones in a slow cooker, and add a little bit of apple cider vinegar or the juice from one lemon, which provides acids in order to extract more nutrients from the bones.

Step 2

Fill the slow cooker with water, and set it to low heat for 24 hours.

Step 3

After the 24 hours, you can flavor your broth with some veggies. Since you won't be consuming these, you may opt to not peel them. Some examples might be onion, celery, and carrots. You can also add parsley, sea salt, and pepper. Then, let it sit for another 12 hours. The more time you let it cook, the more the bones will break down, and the more nutrients are released.

Step 4

After 30 hours or so, you can check the marrow bones to make sure the marrow has fallen out. Sometimes you may have to use a fork to knock out the marrow from the inside. Let it sit for another six hours.

Step 5

After about 36 hours, you can turn off the slow cooker, and let it cool down naturally. Then, skim out the big stuff like the vegetables.

Step 6

Drain the broth through a mesh colander. Store your broth in glass containers in the fridge for about a week or so.

You can freeze your broth if you don't think you will be able to drink it within a week, and it also makes a great stock to cook with.

As the severity of an unhealthy gut varies among people, it is not possible to determine exactly how long it will take for you to heal your gut. However, the process of restoration can begin immediately when you choose fresh and healthy foods over highly-processed and refined alternatives. Your immune system and gut will thank you.

Chapter 9: Healthy Ways to Recover From Metabolic Disorder

Before discussing what metabolic disorders are and healthy approaches that can assist in recovering from them, a true comprehension of the body's metabolism is necessary. Your body uses or receives energy from the food you eat through a process called metabolism. Food is made up of fats, carbohydrates, and proteins—and the chemicals in your digestive system break down these food parts into acids and sugars, your body's fuel. Your body can then either use this fuel right away, or it can store the energy in your fats, muscles, and tissues. Your gut microbiota plays an important part in your metabolism. When abnormal chemical reactions in the body disturb this process, a metabolic disorder occurs. When this happens, you may have too little or too much of certain substances that you need to stay healthy. One can develop a metabolic disorder when certain organs, such as the pancreas or liver, do not function properly or become diseased. Diabetes is a common example of a metabolic disorder.

Metabolic disorders can come in different forms, including:

- A missing vitamin or enzyme that is vital for a certain chemical reaction;
- Nutritional deficiencies;
- Chemical reactions that are abnormal and interfere with metabolic processes; and
- A disease in one of the organs involved in metabolism, including the pancreas, liver, or endocrine glands.

These disorders can develop if certain organs fail to work properly. Sometimes these disorders can be a result of genetics, but in other cases, a person may be deficient in a certain enzyme or hormone, or they could be consuming too much of certain foods, among other factors. There are many genetic metabolic disorders which result from mutations of single genes, and these mutations are inherited and passed down through generations of families.

Diabetes is the most common metabolic disorder, of which there are two types, type 1 and type 2. The cause of type 1 is unknown, although there could be a genetic factor. Type 1 can lead to eyesight impairment, nerve and kidney damage and an increased risk of heart disease. Type 2 can be acquired, but could also be caused by genetic factors as well.

Metabolic Syndrome

One very common metabolic disorder today is called metabolic syndrome, also known as syndrome x. It affects an estimated 40 percent of people over the age of 60. Metabolic syndrome is a term for a cluster of risk factors that can increase your chances of developing heart disease and other health problems. Generally speaking, lack of activity and excess weight can lead to the development of this syndrome, but there five factors specifically that can put you at risk for it.

1. High blood pressure
2. High triglyceride levels
3. High levels of blood sugar
4. Low levels of HDL cholesterol (the good kind)
5. Maintaining a large waistline. This would be more than a 35-inch circumference for women, and more than 40-inch for men.

If you think you may be at a high risk of developing metabolic syndrome based on the five factors listed above, there are measures that you can take to control, prevent or even reverse it. These measures include changes in diet and an increase in exercise. If you don't attempt to make these changes, metabolic syndrome could develop further health risks related to stroke, heart disease, and diabetes. The following are healthy tips for recovering from metabolic syndrome.

Develop a Plant-Based Diet

A plant-based diet can not only help curb metabolic syndrome, but it is also good for your heart. A plant-based diet would showcase veggies, fruits, legumes, and whole grains, and would limit meats and dairy.

Take Note of Your Liquid Intake

Try to avoid sugar-filled beverages and fruit juices, as these can make your triglyceride levels and blood sugar soar. The best option when you are thirsty is to just drink water.

Aim for Healthy Weight Loss

Setting small and specific goals for yourself make weight loss easier. Even losing a little bit of weight can have a significant impact on metabolic syndrome, impacting important numbers like blood sugar, blood pressure, and cholesterol. Remember to set reasonable expectations for yourself, as these are more encouraging.

Avoid Sitting for Long Periods of Time

Sedentary activities that force you to sit, such as watching television, sitting at work and using a computer, have been linked to an increased risk of metabolic syndrome, even if you are exercising regularly.

Stop Smoking

Smoking greatly increases your risk of heart disease, although it is not technically a risk factor for what is known as metabolic syndrome.

Avoid Foods That Aggravate Metabolic Syndrome

All fake foods should be avoided when trying to recover from metabolic syndrome, including processed foods, artificial sweeteners, trans fatty acids (found in foods made with hydrogenated oils and fats, such as margarine, cookies, cakes, pies, crackers and coffee creamers), refined carbohydrates and sugar and alcohol in excess.

Chapter 10: Eating Habits and Foods to Avoid

On the road to a healthy gut and strong immune system, there are a number of foods that can be included in your diet that will benefit and steer you on the right path. There are also many foods that can have extremely damaging effects on your immune system and gut health. These have been touched on in previous chapters but will now be discussed in more detail. You now know that a healthy gut is the foundation of a healthy body. You also know that when your gut microbiota is diverse and balanced, every other part of your body will benefit. Similarly, if your gut flora is out of balance, everything from your mood to your metabolism can be affected. What you eat plays an extremely big role in your gut health. Listed below are many foods that have a high potential to disturb and damage your gut flora.

Artificial Sweeteners

Often times when people are trying to lose weight, they turn to artificial sweeteners, thinking they are healthy because they don't have any calories. However artificial sweeteners can cause changes in your gut microbiota, lead to higher rates of metabolic disorders and increase glucose intolerance.

Processed Foods

Many of us know that processed foods are not healthy, but what may be surprising to you is the effect they can have on the balance of your digestive system. In studies done on mice, it has been shown that the additives used in heavily processed food disrupted their gut microbiota so much that some actually developed metabolic diseases.

Sugar

White refined sugar is not the only sugar that is bad for your health. Sugar in any form can be harmful. People who have a high-sugar diet can experience constipation and overall poor gut function. Some studies have shown that a diet high in sugar causes a change in gut bacteria, impairing the ability to adapt to changing situations. This change in gut bacteria can also have a negative effect on memory. Diets high in fat and sugar disrupt a healthy microbial balance. Sugars are digested easily by us, and they are absorbed by our small intestine without help from our gut microbiota. This leaves our gut bugs hungry with nothing to eat, so they start to nibble on the mucus which lines our intestines. This intestinal lining is meant to be a strong barrier between the gut and the rest of the body, because when it is permeated and particles of food are allowed to enter the bloodstream, what begins to happen? Yes, you are correct, your gut begins to leak.

Gluten

While people suffering from celiac disease are particularly vulnerable to its effects, gluten has also been known to cause stomach pain, fatigue and bloating in those who do not have the disease also.

Grains

While not all grains contain gluten, even gluten-free grains such as brown rice should be avoided while healing your gut. Grains contain phytic acid, a protective coating that can be difficult for the body to digest and break down, resulting in inflammation. Later, after your gut is repaired, you can begin to reintroduce grains slowly.

Soy

Often thought of as beneficial and nutritious, today's soy goes through very high levels of processing. This processing has changed how it affects the body. High levels of soy in your diet can have adverse effects on your gut microbiota as it actually has been shown to reduce levels of healthy bacteria.

Red Meat

Eating red meat encourages the growth of certain bacteria strains that may negatively impact your health, from your immunity to your weight and emotional state. In studies of the microbiota of meat-eaters versus vegetarians, it has been shown that the microbiota of meat-eaters produces more of a certain chemical that is associated with heart disease than does that of vegetarians.

Dairy

Even if you don't suffer from lactose intolerance, large amounts of dairy may not be the best choice for your digestive system. Some studies have shown that consuming dairy changes the microbiota in your gut within days, allowing the bad bacteria, those linked to inflammation and intestinal disease, to flourish.

Genetically-Modified Organisms (GMOs)

In an attempt to grow crops that are naturally resistant to disease and pests, scientists have created genetically-modified organisms (GMOs). GMOs are living organisms whose genetic material has been manipulated artificially through genetic engineering in a laboratory. This creates combinations of plant, bacteria, animal and virus genes that do not naturally exist in nature. Most GMOs have been engineered to tolerate direct application of herbicide. Corn, soybeans, and wheat are the three most common GMOs grown in the United States. The characteristics that allow GMOs to resist disease can wreak havoc on your gut health, reducing the populations of beneficial bacteria.

Farmed Fish

Usually, we think of consuming fish as healthy, and it is, but there is a major distinction between farmed fish and wild-caught fish. Farmed fish can be bad for your gut because of the use of antibiotics in raising them. Huge amounts of antibiotics are added to the food that farmed fish eat, and this can be passed along to humans as the fish are eaten. Any antibiotic that enters the body kills gut bacteria, leading to an unbalanced and unhealthy gut garden.

It is nearly impossible to avoid all of these ingredients all of the time, but taking conscious measures to reduce intake of them can go a long way towards a healthier gut.

Apart from avoiding or completely eliminating certain foods while trying to heal your gut, there are also certain eating habits that can be detrimental to restoration.

Mindless Snacking

Consuming excessive snacks can be dangerous not only for your gut health but for other parts of the body as well. You should be able to last four to six hours between meals without snacking, and at night, you should be able to last 12 hours without waking up to eat.

Stress Eating

Many people turn to food as a distraction when they are stressed, but it is not wise to eat when your body is in this condition. When you are feeling stressed, less blood flows to the stomach, slowing the rate of digestion. As a result, the chances of food fermenting in your stomach become higher, leading to stomach bloating and gas.

Eating Too Many Raw Vegetables (At First)

If you are having gut issues, eating too many raw veggies can cause a reduction in the production of enzymes, altering gut microbiome. Also, digesting too many raw vegetables can be a challenge, leading to bloating and abdominal pain. A solution would be to eat cooked veggies instead, and as your digestion improves, you can slowly start adding more and more raw vegetables.

Chapter 11: Approaches to Tracking Your Success on the Road to Recovery

In many cases, the road to a healthy gut can be a long one, but just knowing that you are making improvements is sometimes all the motivation you need to go on. You have already taken many important steps towards recovery. You have followed diet recommendations, such as planning healthy meals, eliminating many unhealthy foods, and adding new and beneficial foods to your daily routine. You have taken measures to eliminate stress, such as getting more sleep and exercising regularly. You have made a more conscious effort to think about what the food you are eating actually does to your body. You will eventually reach a point when you ask yourself, "Is my gut repaired?" Although everyone is different and that it is impossible to determine exactly how long it will take to heal your unhealthy gut, listed below are things to look for when tracking success on your personal road to recovery. If you experience these changes in your body, it is a good sign that you are experiencing a successful recovery from an unhealthy gut.

Food Sensitivities Disappear

If your intestinal wall was weak (your gut was leaking) there is a high chance that you were also sensitive to many foods. One way to track your success is by noticing that you are able to eat foods that previously gave you digestive discomforts, such as headaches, fatigue and mood issues. You will then be able to add more of a variety to your diet and reintroduce healthy foods. Once you have restored good bacteria in your gut it is crucial that you continue to follow a healthy eating plan and keep up good habits. Now that you have attained your goal of improving your gut microbiota, your next goal should be to maintain its health and vitality. After all that hard work, you don't want to experience the same problems all over again.

You No Longer Experience Digestive Issues

Many people who are experiencing gut health issues such as leaky gut suffer symptoms including stomach bloating, acid reflux, gas, heartburn, and constipation. When these burdens start to go away and stay away, it is a positive indicator that your restoration efforts have been paying off.

You Return to Your Ideal Self

A good way to track success on your gut healing journey is to ask yourself whether or not you feel like your "normal self" again. When the microbiota of your gut is unbalanced, you are very likely living with symptoms that are affecting the quality of your life in some way. A good indication that the bacteria in your gut have become balanced is that your energy has returned, you experience improvements in your mood, you notice better mental clarity, you have reached a healthy weight, you experience less stress and you just feel like yourself again.

As mentioned in other chapters, stress plays an important part in gut health. During times of stress, blood flow to the digestive system becomes restricted, altering the bacteria in your gut, causing issues like low energy and unpleasant mood. Due to the communication between the gut and the brain and their complex relationship, when your gut bacteria are unbalanced, it becomes difficult to handle stressful situations. Because of this two-way street, restoring your unhealthy gut allows you to feel less stress. If you are noticing that you are less stressed out than you used to be, good job, you are healing your gut. Ensuring that you are exercising regularly and getting enough sleep will also help manage stress.

It is important to know that gut health is on a spectrum. On one end you have a completely healthy gut, living with no symptoms. On the other end, you have many symptoms, a leaky gut and may even be on your way to being diagnosed with an autoimmune disease. If you are at this end, repairing your gut will move you back down the spectrum and you will notice improvements along the way. During your restoration, however, you may experience incidents or setbacks that move you back up the spectrum. These setbacks could include contracting an infection while traveling, the need to take antibiotics or an accidental gluten exposure. In any of these cases, you will need to work your way back down the spectrum again.

Skin Issues Go Away

Many skin conditions, such as rosacea, acne, rashes, dandruff, and eczema, are the body's outward expression of an internal problem related to your gut microbiota and immune system. If your skin issues are subsiding, it is a good indication that your gut is being repaired.

Your Autoimmune Lab Results Improve

As your immune system is impacted greatly by your gut health, restoring your gut often leads to an improvement in various autoimmune lab indicators. Many patients will notice that their lab results have improved, often seeing their antibodies go negative. This is a good sign that your gut flora is becoming more diversified.

As you boost your immune system through better gut health, you may also notice other changes in your body—such as a decrease in colds and the time they stick around. We all catch colds once in a while, but if your colds seem to last a long time and are followed by cold after cold, it is likely your immune system is not functioning as it should, and something is wrong with your gut as well. Improving gut health allows you to build a strong immune system, preventing harmful bugs from entering your body. It may help to imagine your immune system as a fortress. When the door of the fortress is open, invaders can easily enter. Through healing your gut and, in turn, boosting your immune system, you are closing the door to the fortress, making it more difficult for unwanted intruders to pass through.

You can use the previously listed indicators to track how successful you are in your goal of attaining a healthy gut. They all involve listening to your body and becoming more aware of what it is trying to tell you. Becoming more mindful of your body is essential to overall health and well-being.

Conclusion

Thanks for making it through to the end of *Immune System: Boost the Immune System, Heal Your Gut, and Cleanse Your Body Naturally*. Let's hope it was informative and provided you with all of the tools you need to achieve your goals. Many people today are suffering from problems related to gut health, which affects how the immune system functions. If you have read this book, you may only be interested in learning more about having a healthy gut microbiota and staying healthy. On the other hand, you might be aiming to heal an unhealthy gut and looking for tips on how to start the journey towards restoration.

The first step in your recovery process is simply realizing that it is possible to boost your immune system and heal your gut naturally. It is then important to understand how these two systems, immune and digestive, work together and affect each other. There are so many benefits of having a healthy immune system and gut, and the sooner you begin your personal recovery process, the sooner you will reap these rewards. People have problems with their immune system for various reasons, but many of these issues can be dealt with by first focusing on your gut. By following the very doable suggestions in this book, you will be very well on your way to optimal gut health in no time. However, before setting off on the road to recovery, take a personal inventory of your own immune system and gut health, and take note of what issues you may have. Listen to your body, and try to understand what it is telling you. After doing this, it will be time to set goals and start your journey towards healing your unhealthy gut—and your immune system will thank you. Remember to set small, attainable goals, as they tend to be more motivating and encouraging.

With your goals set, you can start taking the necessary measures outlined in this book and head off on your trip to gut health. Take into consideration the healthy diets recommended in chapter six. Add foods to your shopping list, which will boost your immune system and improve the bacterial balance in your gut. Take the time to plan healthy meals, and remember to eat a wide variety of foods in order to diversify your gut microbiota. Even though it may seem difficult at first, the planning of nourishing, gut healthy meals will get easier. As you start to heal your gut and feel better, you will be encouraged to continue your new diet habits. As you now know what foods to avoid, you will witness the wide array of benefits that can be received from eliminating them from your diet. After all of your hard work and dedication towards gut restoration, you will, of course, want to know if it has all been worth it, and the final chapter of this book provides ways to track gut recovery success.